23 Low-Impact Workouts to Build Stronger
Knees, Ease Pain, and Get You Moving
Again in Just 10 Minutes a Day

KNEE
STRENGTHENING
AND STRETCHING
EXERCISES
FOR SENIORS

Ottie Oz

Table of Content

Ready to enhance your fitness journey?

Simply scan the QR code or enter the URL to download exclusive access to our transformative health resources!

You'll get **Extra Core Exercises**, featuring **six meticulously organized routines** to strengthen your core, a **Knee Exercises Tracker** to monitor your progress and maximize results, and **Wrist Routines** designed to maintain joint health. Don't wait—**take the first step towards a stronger, healthier you today!**

https://books.bookfunnel.com/kneestrengthening

Introduction

It's never too late to take your first step toward wellness.
– J a n e   F o n d a

We live in a world that is constantly evolving, and one of the most positive shifts in recent years has been the growing interest in longevity and healthy aging. Seniors today are more focused than ever on leading active and fulfilling lives well into their golden years.

Current statistics highlight that over 750 million people worldwide are now aged 65 or older (United Nations, 2022)—the highest number in history and nearly six times more than in 1950. Back in 1950, global life expectancy averaged just 47 years. Today, it's risen to 71 years (Dattani et al., 2023). Someone born 70 years ago witnessed a world without widespread telephones or televisions, before space exploration, computers, the internet, or mobile phones. Meanwhile, a child born today is almost certain to see the 22nd century.

This rise in life expectancy and the growing number of older adults can be attributed to several factors, one of which is the push towards more active lifestyles. For many seniors, staying active isn't a new concept—they grew up in an era when outdoor play was the norm and movement was a natural part of daily life. However, what might have changed over the years is the ease with which these activities can be done. As we age, certain physical activities may become more challenging, and for some, even simple tasks like getting out of bed or maintaining balance can be difficult.

Fortunately, advancements in understanding how the body ages and methods to maintain muscle strength and joint health mean that the challenges of aging don't have to define your future. What if you could maintain or even improve your knee health using something as simple as an everyday chair?

In this guide, we'll explore how knee exercises designed for seniors can be easily performed with or without the support of a chair. These targeted exercises can help rebuild muscle strength, improve balance, and boost your confidence, leading to an enhanced quality of life. We'll delve into the benefits of staying active as you age, provide step-by-step instructions for effective knee exercises, and guide you in building a sustainable exercise routine. The goal is to empower you with the tools you need to maintain mobility, manage weight, and enjoy life to the fullest.

Keeping Your Knees in the Game: What You Need to Know

Our knees are nothing short of amazing. Our knees are the silent heroes behind every walk, squat, and stretch. They help us stay mobile and independent. Sure, they might start to creak or need a little extra care, but they're far from finished.

They're more than simple hinges—they're well-coordinated teams, built from cartilage, ligaments, tendons, and even a little natural lubrication. Each part has a job to keep us gliding through life, but with time, the game changes. Cartilage might wear thin, ligaments lose their spring, and the synovial fluid that kept things running smoothly isn't as plentiful as it used to be. But understanding these shifts isn't about worrying—it's about knowing exactly how to give our knees the support they deserve as they age gracefully along with us. So, shall we take a closer look at how our knees are constructed and how they evolve over time?

- **Cartilage**: This cushioning allows us to move pain-free, but it does thin over time, sometimes leading to stiffness or discomfort (American Academy of Orthopaedic Surgeons, 2021). With age, the body's ability to repair cartilage slows down, leading to "bone-on-bone" friction and pain. This thinning is a primary reason for the high rates of osteoarthritis in older adults (National Institute of Arthritis and Musculoskeletal and Skin Diseases, 2018).

- **Ligaments**: These bands hold the knee steady, but as we age, they lose some elasticity, increasing the risk of sprains and instability (Mayo Clinic, 2022).

- **Muscle Weakness**: The muscles surrounding the knee, like the quadriceps and hamstrings, naturally lose strength over time. This decline places extra pressure on the knee joint, which can lead to additional discomfort or pain (Mayo Clinic, 2022).

- **Bone Density Loss**: Many people experience a decrease in bone density as they age, a condition known as osteoporosis. Weaker bones provide less protection for the knee joint, increasing the risk of fractures and injuries (National Institute on Aging, 2020).

- **Tendons**: These connect muscles to bones and are essential for all movement. However, tendons also weaken over time, which can limit mobility and make simple movements feel more challenging (National Institute on Aging, 2020).

- **Synovial Fluid**: This natural lubricant allows for smooth, pain-free movement in the knee joint. Unfortunately, as we get older, the body produces less synovial fluid, which can lead to stiffness—especially in the morning or after sitting for long periods (Arthritis Foundation, 2019).

The Realities of Knee Health with Age

For many of us, knee pain is not just a possibility—it's a guarantee. The years of moving, bending, lifting, and standing accumulate, and aging brings additional hurdles. However, the encouraging news is that while we can't turn back time, we can absolutely prioritize our knee health starting today. We don't have to let knee discomfort dictate our lives. With intentional effort, we can take control, alleviate the pain, and embrace a life filled with strength and vitality. Let's make our knees a priority and keep moving forward!

Let's look at the most common knee concerns we encounter as we age:

- **Osteoarthritis:** Often called "wear-and-tear" arthritis, osteoarthritis occurs when the cartilage around the knee wears away over time. This can lead to pain, swelling, and reduced range of motion, making everyday tasks like walking or bending more difficult (Johns Hopkins Medicine, 2022).

- **Patellar Tendinitis:** Also known as "jumper's knee," patellar tendinitis occurs when the tendons that link the kneecap to the shin become inflamed. Though it often comes from sports, repetitive strain on weakened tendons can bring on this condition in older adults, too (Cleveland Clinic, 2021).

🌿 **Bursitis:** Small, fluid-filled sacs around the knee that help reduce friction. However, with age or repeated pressure, these sacs can become irritated, causing pain and swelling—a condition known as bursitis (American College of Rheumatology, 2020).

🌿 **Ligament Laxity and Weakness:** Ligaments are strong bands that keep our knees stable, but as we age, they stretch out and lose some strength. This can make our knees less stable, increasing the risk of falls or injuries from even simple movements (Centers for Disease Control and Prevention, 2021).

Proactive Knee Care for Lifelong Mobility

While aging does bring a few unavoidable changes, it's never too late to adopt habits that help our knees feel younger, stronger, and ready for action. Here are four key strategies to keep those knees in top shape as we move through life:

- **Regular Low-Impact Exercise:** Research shows that regular physical activity—especially low-impact exercises like walking, swimming, and cycling—does wonders for knee health. These activities enhance knee function, reduce pain, and can even slow arthritis progression. (Harvard Health Publishing, 2019). Keeping our knees healthy is like maintaining a well-tuned car. Just as regular oil changes and gentle drives keep the engine running smoothly, low-impact exercises and mindful movement help our knees function at their best. Neglecting either can lead to unexpected issues down the road.

- **Maintaining a Healthy Weight:** Every extra pound adds about four pounds of pressure on the knees (imagine them saying, "Whoa there!"), especially during activities like walking or climbing stairs. Studies reveal that even modest weight loss can make a big difference, reducing knee pain and improving function. In fact, losing as little as 5% of body weight can yield impressive benefits for knee health (Arthritis Foundation, 2019).

- **Nutrient-Rich Diet:** Think of certain nutrients as a VIP pass for your joints. Omega-3 fatty acids from salmon and other fish help reduce inflammation, while calcium and vitamin D keep bones dense and strong. And don't forget those colorful fruits and veggies—they're packed with antioxidants that help protect joint tissues from wear and tear (American Academy of Orthopaedic Surgeons, 2021).

- **Supportive Footwear and Orthotics:** Don't underestimate the power of good shoes! The right footwear, especially with orthotic inserts, can provide stability and alignment. It helps to alleviate knee strain by keeping posture in check and reducing joint stress. It's like a little hug for your knees every time you take a step (Cleveland Clinic, 2021).

Let's not allow pain and limited mobility to dictate our ability to engage in the activities we love. It's important to understand how our knees change with age, and with that knowledge, we can take decisive action to keep them strong and capable. By prioritizing our knee health, we can ensure they are always prepared to support us in every challenge and adventure ahead. This book offers exercises designed to support and strengthen your knees, so you can keep moving with confidence and independence. Remember, each small step towards better knee health is a step towards a fuller and more enjoyable life!

If you're still not convinced about starting to exercise, then shall we take a look at how strengthening your leg muscles can help your knees feel better.

The Benefits of Knee Strengthening Exercises

Taking charge of your knee health through strengthening exercises is not just about reducing discomfort—it's a declaration of independence over the movements that shape your day. Strengthen those muscles, and you're essentially giving your knees a team of bodyguards—ones that absorb impact and keep everything moving smoothly. These exercises are more than just routines; they're your way of reclaiming confidence and moving with purpose. Why should you settle for shuffling steps when you can stride with power? Dive in, and let's talk about how strengthening your knees can turbocharge your mobility, balance, and overall well-being.

- **Strengthening Supporting Muscles:** Here's the deal: your knees don't work solo. They're backed by the mighty quadriceps, hamstrings, glutes, and calves. Think of these as the A-team that holds it all together. Strong quadriceps stabilize the kneecap like a well-oiled hinge, while your hamstrings take on the role of shock absorbers, easing the strain on your knee joint with each step (American Academy of Orthopaedic Surgeons, 2021). It's like equipping your legs with their own built-in suspension system.

Promoting Better Joint Alignment: Alignment isn't just for cars; your knees need it too. Strengthening exercises help keep the knee joint aligned, reducing pressure on the cartilage and ligaments. The result? Less wear and tear, fewer chances of creaks and cracks that slow you down. Simple moves like squats and leg raises do wonders for muscle alignment—it's all about keeping those parts working in harmony (Cleveland Clinic, 2022). Who says aging has to come with a side of stiffness?

Enhancing Knee Stability: Stability—that's the secret sauce to knees that doesn't betray you with a sudden buckle or twist. As we age, ligaments lose some of their elasticity, but targeted exercises can help turn the tide. Whether it's standing leg lifts or resistance band workouts, these moves reinforce the ligaments and create a strong "support network" for your knees. When your knees are fortified, they're less likely to give out, turning falls and injuries into a distant memory (National Institute on Aging, 2021).

Building a Support Network for Your Knees: Strengthening exercises aren't just about flexing your muscles; they're about crafting a support network that takes the load off the joint itself. This shift in burden means your knees can keep working smoothly without crying for mercy. Over time, this leads to more ease, more confidence, and more "yes" to the activities you love.

So go ahead, channel that spirit of playful defiance. Squash the myth that aging means slowing down. Your knees are more capable than they've been given credit for, and with the right moves, they'll prove that there's still rocket fuel in the tanks of those who've weathered a few seasons.

❧ **Increased Range of Motion:** Think of your knees as hinges that deserve a little TLC to keep them swinging smoothly. Strengthening exercises are your maintenance plan, helping preserve and even improve that range of motion. Over time, muscles and tendons can tighten like an old rubber band, restricting movement. But with exercises like calf raises or hamstring curls, you can stretch and strengthen those muscles, letting you move with the kind of fluidity that keeps life from slowing down (Johns Hopkins Medicine, 2020).

❧ **Enhanced Balance and Coordination:** Balance is more than just a party trick; it's what keeps you confident and steady on your feet. Exercises like single-leg stands or step-ups train not just the knee but the entire team—core, hips, and all—to work together seamlessly. This coordination is your insurance against stumbles and falls, a common worry for many seniors. Strong knee muscles mean better stability and a sense of control, letting you move with confidence. Research backs it up: leg-strengthening exercises improve postural stability, making you feel secure in your movements (Harvard Health Publishing, 2019).

- **Positive Impact on Daily Functionality:** Have you ever struggled to get up from a chair or climb a flight of stairs without feeling like you're scaling Everest? Strengthened knees can make these everyday tasks feel like a breeze. By fortifying the knee and surrounding muscles, you're reducing the effort needed for these activities. Less effort means less fatigue, which translates to more energy for doing the things you love—be it gardening, walking, or playing with the grandkids (American Geriatrics Society, 2021).

- **Quality of Life Boost:** Enhanced mobility and balance aren't just nice-to-haves—they're life changers. Think of what it means to join a friend for a walk, spend a sunny afternoon lost in your garden, or chase after your grandkids with ease and joy. When you don't have to second-guess every step or worry about a stumble, you gain more than just physical freedom—you gain the confidence that spills into every part of your day. The ability to move without fear isn't just about comfort; it's about living fully, with a smile that comes from the inside out.

- **Pain Reduction and Improved Joint Comfort:** One of the biggest wins from knee-strengthening exercises? Less pain. Chronic knee pain can trick you into moving less, setting off a chain reaction where less movement leads to more stiffness and discomfort. But here's the truth: you can break that cycle. With the right exercises, relief isn't just possible—it's within reach.

- **Reducing Strain on the Knee Joint:** Let's put it this way: when your muscles step up, your joints get to take a well-deserved break. Strengthening exercises let your muscles take on more of the load so that your knee joint isn't working overtime. Strong quadriceps, for instance, act like shock absorbers, handling the impact of walking and standing and giving your knee joint a bit of a breather. For anyone navigating arthritis or joint wear and tear, this kind of muscle support can slow down cartilage loss and make daily life feel easier (Arthritis Foundation, 2020).

- **Alleviating Inflammation and Swelling:** It might seem odd to move when you're in pain, but movement is actually your ally. Gentle, low-impact exercises—think easy squats or leg raises—get your blood flowing, which helps cut down on inflammation and swelling. And it's not just wishful thinking; science backs it up. Regular movement improves circulation, which in turn eases pain and helps soothe inflamed joints (Mayo Clinic, 2021).

- **Improving Joint Lubrication:** As we get older, that smooth, comfortable joint movement we once took for granted can start to feel like a thing of the past. The natural production of synovial fluid—the body's joint lubricant—slows down, making knees stiffer and movements less fluid. But there's good news: movement can kickstart this process. Simple exercises that involve bending and extending the knee can spark the release of synovial fluid, helping to coat and cushion the joint, easing friction, and bringing much-needed relief from stiffness (National Institute of Arthritis and Musculoskeletal and Skin Diseases, 2020). If your knees have been giving you that telltale "creak", it's time to get them moving and greased up.

Supporting Mental Health and Pain Relief. Pain doesn't just stay in the knees; it seeps into your mindset, affecting mood and day-to-day joy. The frustration, sadness, and isolation that come with chronic pain are real and can be tough to shake. But regular exercise isn't just a remedy for the body—it's a tonic for the mind. Movement releases endorphins, nature's built-in mood lifters, which help fend off anxiety and depression. The best part? The relief you feel from stronger, healthier knees doesn't just stay physical; it builds a sense of accomplishment that can brighten your mood and keep you looking forward with hope (American Psychological Association, 2019).

The benefits of knee-strengthening exercises reach far beyond just easing pain. They help build emotional strength and resilience, giving you the confidence to step out, engage with the world, and approach each day with a sense of renewed optimism and vigor.

You don't have to get caught up in routines or spend hours on end exercising—incorporating a few movements into your daily routine can go a long way in promoting knee health and happiness effortlessly! The routines included in this book are designed to be completed in just 10–15 minutes a day. It's not that much and you don't need fancy clothes or equipment to do so. You will stick to the routines you will notice the improvement. Maybe not overnight though but you will.

This is why it's important to be realistic and set realistic goals.

Setting Realistic Goals

Embarking on the path to stronger knees is empowering, especially when you set goals that are simple, safe, and motivating. Forget complicated plans—the best goals are the ones that fit into your life and make progress feel rewarding. Here's how to set goals that inspire, keep you safe, and make every small victory count.

Creating Goals That Motivate and Inspire

Start by thinking about what really matters to you. Maybe you want to walk without that nagging discomfort, climb stairs without hesitation, or simply feel more confident in your daily movements. When your goals have a personal meaning, each exercise becomes more than just a task—it becomes a step toward reclaiming the moments that make life enjoyable.

Break your goals down into short-term and long-term achievements. Start with something small and doable, like "I'll do my knee exercises three times a week for 10 minutes." Small wins build momentum, and over time, these efforts add up. Before you know it, that short-term goal can evolve into bigger milestones, like taking the stairs without a second thought or strolling around the block comfortably. Remember, progress is progress, no matter how small.

Practical Tip: Start with a 4-Week Plan

Create a schedule tha   t includes three 10–15-minute sessions per week focused on knee-strengthening exercises. You have plenty of routines to choose from in this book; from very basic to more challenging. Download the progress tracker and record your progress. Alternatively, you can use any journal to record your progress. Keeping track of your progress can be incredibly motivating. Every small gain adds up, and noting these changes can keep you committed. A simple journal works wonders—jot down the exercises you did, how you felt afterward, and any shifts in comfort or strength. It's a way to look back and see how far you've come.

At the beginning of this book, you'll find a QR code and link. When you scan or enter it, you'll gain access to extra materials designed to enhance your knee-strengthening experience. This includes a collection of core exercises along with five additional routines specifically tailored to help strengthen your core and complement the knee exercises in this book.

After four weeks, check in with yourself to see how you're doing and tweak your routine as needed.

Prioritizing Safety at Every Step

If you're new to exercise or managing knee pain, safety comes first. Start slow, listen to your body, and remember: there's a difference between the healthy fatigue of working muscles and sharp pain that signals trouble. If you have any health concerns, it might be best to consult your doctor or a physician before you start. While most older adults should be able to complete these exercises without problems, there are certain situations where certain individuals might not be able to do them.

Practical Tip: Use Mirrors or Support for Better Form

Using a mirror helps you see if you're maintaining good form, like keeping your knees behind your toes during mini-squats or ensuring your back stays straight. If you need a little extra stability, holding onto a chair for support lets you focus on moving confidently.

Finding Joy in the Process

Setting knee health goals isn't just about the result—it's about enjoying the journey. Each small step forward, whether it's feeling a little stronger or noticing less pain, matters. Be patient with yourself. Some days will be tougher than others, and that's okay. What counts is showing up and making an effort.

Find ways to make the process enjoyable. Listen to your favorite music, share your progress with loved ones, or work out with a friend. Adding a social element can make all the difference, turning exercise into a shared and uplifting experience. And when you hit a milestone, take time to celebrate. Treat yourself to something special, like a good book or a relaxing day out.

Practical Tip: Celebrate Milestones

Reward yourself for meeting your goals. After a month of consistent exercise, treat yourself—maybe a new book, a relaxing massage, or a piece of equipment that makes your routine more enjoyable. These small rewards add a touch of fun and recognition to your hard work.

Reflecting on the Benefits

When you look back at what you've achieved, you'll see that the benefits go beyond the physical. Stronger knees mean less pain and more ease, but they also mean a more confident, independent you. You might find that you feel prouder, more optimistic, and ready to tackle whatever comes next.

Remember, every bit of effort you put in now is an investment in your future comfort, mobility, and independence. Each small gain in strength and flexibility is a step toward more freedom in your daily life. So here's to setting goals that are meaningful to you and taking each step forward with pride and confidence. Keep moving, keep celebrating, and know that every effort counts.

Tips on How to Incorporate Knee Exercises into Daily Life

Making knee exercises a part of your daily routine doesn't have to be a burden. Mixing strengthening movements with daily activities allows you to create a routine that feels simple, manageable, and enjoyable. Here's how to make knee exercises a natural part of your life, overcome common challenges, and adjust your routine as your strength builds.

- **Making Exercise Part of Your Routine:** The easiest way to build an exercise habit is to weave it into what you're already doing. That way, it doesn't feel like a separate task demanding time you don't have.

- **Exercises While Waiting:** Don't let those idle moments go to waste. Use the time you spend waiting for the coffee to brew or brushing your teeth to fit in some standing exercises. Calf raises are quick and effective: just lift onto the balls of your feet, hold for a second, and slowly lower back down. If you're near a sturdy surface, mini squats are another great choice. These small movements engage the muscles around your knees. It makes them stronger without taking up extra time.

- **During Screen Time:** Sneak in some knee-friendly moves while sitting at your PC or watching TV. Seated knee extensions are easy: extend one leg out straight, tighten your thigh, and hold for a few seconds before lowering. This simple exercise strengthens your quadriceps, which are crucial for knee stability. You can also try heel slides—gently slide one foot back toward the chair to bend the knee. These subtle movements keep your knees active, even when you're sitting.

Finding Joy in Movement: Who says exercise has to be a grind? Rediscovering the simple pleasures of movement can be the secret to stronger knees and a happier heart. Whether it's tending to your garden, dancing in your living room, or going for a stroll with friends, these activities do more than just keep you active—they remind you that movement is meant to be enjoyed. And here's the best part: while you're laughing, chatting, and moving, your knees are reaping the benefits. Natural, fluid movements support joint health and strengthen the muscles around your knees, all while boosting your mood and nurturing social connections—a win for body, mind, and spirit (National Institute on Aging, 2021).

Overcoming Common Barriers: Starting and maintaining a new exercise routine isn't always smooth sailing. Sometimes life throws in expected events in your way, such as lack of time, motivation dips, or initial discomfort. Here's how to tackle some of these common challenges head-on:

🌿 **Limited Time:** Finding a large block of time to exercise can feel next to impossible some days. But here's the good news: you don't need it. Routines in this book take only 10-15 minutes to perform. You can also select individual exercises and repeat them throughout the day. Any movement is better than none. Even five-minute stretches in the morning or while you're watching TV can make a noticeable difference. The key is consistency over duration—short but regular sessions will gradually build your strength and become part of your day without feeling overwhelmed.

🌿 **Managing Discomfort:** If you're dealing with discomfort, starting with gentle movements and making modifications can help ease you in. Try warming up with a warm compress on your knees to reduce stiffness and make movement easier. Always listen to your body; if an exercise feels too intense or causes pain, scale it back or modify it to suit your comfort level. Remind yourself constantly that building knee strength is a marathon, not a sprint. Focus on making progress that feels sustainable.

🌿 **Staying Motivated:** Keeping your motivation up can be tricky, but finding ways to make exercises enjoyable will keep you going. Pair knee exercises with something you love, like listening to a favorite podcast or show, to make the routine feel more like a well-deserved break than a task. Tracking your progress also helps; even small wins, like feeling less stiffness or moving more easily, remind you why you're doing this and keep you inspired to stick with it.

- **Building a Support System:** Everything's better with a buddy. If you have friends or family members, ask if they would join you. Doing exercises together adds a fun, social aspect to your routine and keeps you both accountable. Plus, sharing the journey makes it more enjoyable and helps push you through the tougher days.

- **Increasing Exercises Difficulty when You Improve:** As you keep up with your knee exercises, you'll start noticing improvements in strength and comfort. To stay motivated and continue progressing, it's important to keep your routine fresh and challenging.

If you will stick to being consistent with exercises the day will come that the exercises that you found difficult before are fairly easy or too easy to complete. You'll notice you need less of your chair support or can do more repetitions. This is when you will know it's time to raise the bar. Adding a few more repetitions or an extra set can keep your muscles engaged and help you build more strength. For example, if you've been doing 10 seated leg lifts, try increasing it up to 15 repetitions per leg. These small things keep your muscles guessing and working harder.

- **Introducing Balance Exercises.** As your muscle strength improves, add balance exercises into the routine.

It can bring a new level of challenge and strengthen the stabilizing muscles around the knee. Try a single-leg stand by holding onto a sturdy surface and balancing on one leg for a few seconds. Exercises like these increase coordination and support knee stability, preparing you for everyday movements with more confidence.

- **Take Exercises Outside.** When the weather is nice, consider doing your knee exercises outside. A change of scenery, like a park or your backyard, can lift your spirits and make the exercises feel more like an enjoyable activity than a task. Fresh air can do wonders for your mood and energy.

- **A Lifestyle of Strength and Mobility.** Incorporating knee exercises into your daily life isn't just about building strength; it's about crafting a lifestyle that supports your health, mobility, and independence. Making these exercises part of your day sets you up for benefits that go beyond physical strength—it makes everyday activities easier and more comfortable.

The key as in everything is consistency and patience. Each small effort, from morning stretches to mini squats, adds up over time to create a stronger, more resilient body. If you stick to it, you will notice the improvement.

So keep moving forward, and celebrate every step along the way. You're building a routine that prioritizes your well-being and supports a healthier, more active life—one that allows you to keep doing the things you love with confidence and ease.

Knee health isn't just about walking or bending without wincing—it's about how you engage with life. When your knees are strong and steady, you're not just moving more easily; you're moving with confidence. Suddenly, that trip to the park, playing with the grandkids, or dancing at a family gathering feels less like a challenge and more like a celebration. Every strengthening exercise you do is more than a physical movement—it's a step toward a life that feels fuller and more energized.

Building knee strength isn't just a routine; it's an investment in your independence. With patience and consistency, those small daily efforts add up. They create a foundation that lets you live life on your own terms—with the energy, freedom, and self-assurance you've earned. So, keep going, celebrate every bit of progress, and embrace the journey to a future where your knees keep up with your zest for life.

Getting Ready for Your Exercises

Courage doesn't always roar. Sometimes courage is the quiet voice at the end of the day saying, 'I will try again tomorrow.

– Mary Anne Radmacher

Always start with a warm-up. You can use the one included in this book. If you're already familiar with the exercise world, you then might remember and have practised some exercise in the past. Exercises such as neck rolls arm circles, marching, or running on the spot or in the chair, they're great exercises to use to warm your body and mind up.

At the back of the book, you'll find routines created for your convenience, complete with pictures and suggested repetitions.

Most of the exercises are straightforward, but if you're unfamiliar with them, it's helpful to review the instructions to ensure correct form. Once you're comfortable, you can move on to the routines at the end of the book. The initial routines are basic and ideal for beginners. If you find them easy, consider increasing the repetitions or trying other exercises to see what works best for you. Remember to listen to your body: if the first routine feels challenging, stick with it until you notice improvement. Progress can take time, especially as we age, but consistency is key.

As you build confidence, feel free to create your own routines or spread exercises throughout the day. If you own any of my other books, try mixing exercises to create customized routines. This book alone contains enough exercises to strengthen not only your leg muscles—important for knee health—but also your core, which supports overall health and stability.

Before You Get Started

If you have any health concerns, it's best to consult your doctor or physician before starting. While most older adults should be able to do these exercises without issues, certain individuals may need to take precautions.

- **Clothing:** You don't need special clothing—any comfortable clothes that allow freedom of movement will work fine. However, you will need a sturdy chair for support. Choose a chair without arms to allow greater movement flexibility. The key is to select a chair that stays stable during your exercises. Avoid folding chairs or those with wheels, as they can be unsafe.

- **Equipment:** Some core exercises may need to be performed on the floor. A yoga mat can be helpful if you have hard flooring at home. Also, use your stairs if you have them, or alternatively, a small step or a thick book or two. Just make sure that they don't slide, they're sturdy enough for you to step onto them. If you don't have it, don't worry, there are plenty of exercises to choose from to strengthen your muscles.

- **How Long to Exercise:** People often ask how frequently they should perform the exercises to see results. Since these routines are short—10–15 minutes—it's advisable to do them at least three times a week for better results. However, you can do them daily if you prefer. As mentioned, you can also choose a few exercises and repeat them throughout the day. For example, one day you might do a full routine, the next day spread out 90 leg curls, and on another day, dedicate time to stretching your knees for improved flexibility. Remember, even doing just one or two exercises is much better than doing none at all—every bit of movement counts and makes a difference! It all depends on your current fitness level. Take a look at the exercises and routines to find what suits you best—this is a tool for you to adapt to your lifestyle.

Now that you're all set, make sure your workout area is free of sharp objects and anything that could interfere with your routine or pose a risk of injury. Ensure the space is tidy and calming to avoid distractions. With everything in place, you can start planning your first knee strengthening exercise session.

Warm-Up

The warm-ups prepare the body to exercise. It increases blood flow, warms the muscles, and makes them more flexible.

Neck Stretch

Keep your chin slightly tucked in. Gently turn your head to the right and then to the left. Hold the stretch for 2-3 seconds before moving your head to the opposite side. Repeat the same, moving your head up and down. Repeat 3 times in each direction—left, right, up, and down.

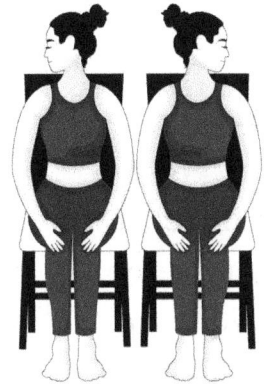

Shoulder Stretch

Bring your hands behind the head. Pull your elbows back as much as possible. Imagine your shoulder blades meeting together. Then, slowly move your elbows forward, trying to touch each other. Repeat the movement 3-5 times.

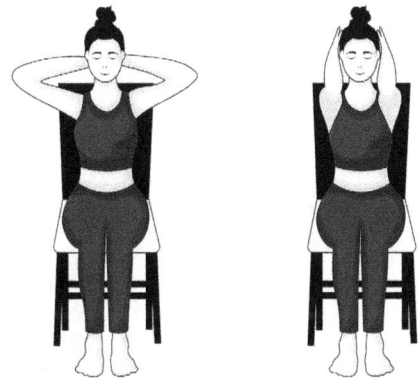

Straight Arm Front Raises

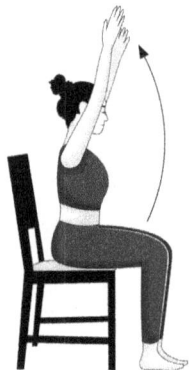

Raise your arms in front of you and lift them above your head, then lower them back down. Repeat this movement 8–10 times.

Run on the Spot

Instead of marching, try running in place as fast as you can for 30 seconds. You can do this either standing or sitting.

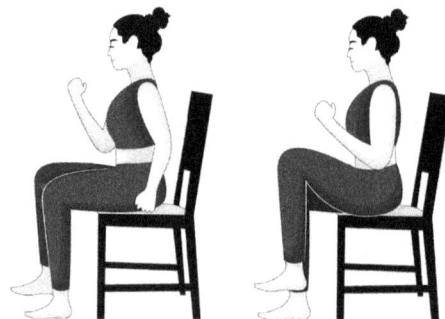

Forward Fold

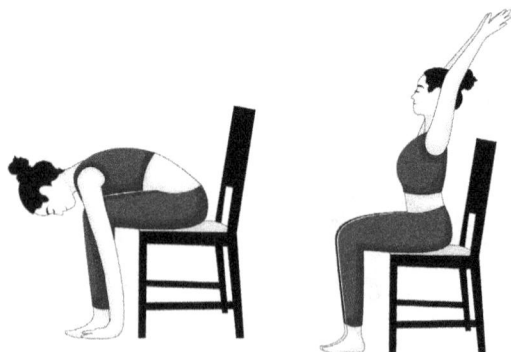

Inhale as you raise your arms for a gentle stretch. Exhale and lower your arms toward your feet, resting your torso on your thighs with your chin close to your knees. **Note:** If you have high blood pressure or find it difficult to breathe, you should not do this pose.

Knee Strengthening Exercises

Standing Hamstring Curls

Instructions: Stand behind a sturdy chair, holding onto the backrest for balance.

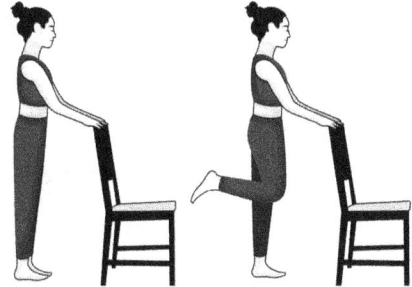

Tighten your core, then bend your right knee to lift your heel toward your glutes, forming a 90-degree angle. Slowly lower your foot back to the floor with control.

Repetitions: Repeat 10-15 times on each leg, then switch. Aim to complete 3 sets.

Sit to Stand

Instructions: Sit near the edge of a sturdy chair, with feet hip-width apart and flat on the floor. Keeping your chest upright, press down through your heels to stand up slowly. Control your descent as you sit back down, aiming to keep your knees behind your toes. Focus on shifting your weight back into the chair without allowing your knees to extend forward.

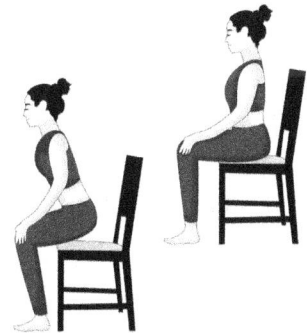

Repetitions: Aim for 8–10 repetitions. Complete 3 sets if comfortable.

Single Leg Quad Sets

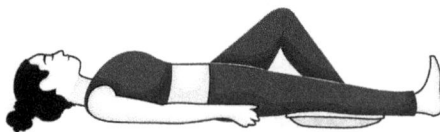

Instructions: Lie down on the floor with your legs extended. Place a pillow lengthwise under your knee. Pull your toes toward yourself and push your leg down to squash the pillow. Hold for 10 seconds and repeat up to 20 times. You should feel your thigh and gluteus muscles during this exercise.

Repetitions: Perform 8-12 repetitions on each leg, then switch. Aim for 3 sets.

Prone Hamstring Curl

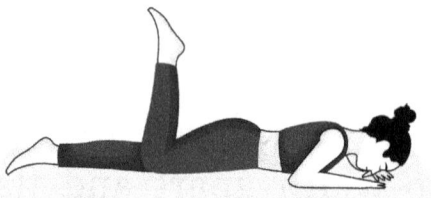

Instructions: Lie down on your stomach and fold your arms in front of you. Bend your knee and move your heel toward your butt. Return to starting position.

Repetitions: Repeat 10–15 times per leg, aiming for 3 sets.

Wall Slides

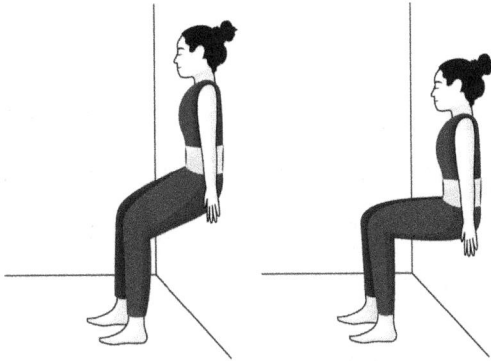

Instructions: Stand with your back, shoulders, and hips against a wall, feet hip-width apart. Step forward 6 – 12 inches from the wall.

Slowly slide down into a squat, keeping your knees over your ankles. Hold briefly, then slide back up in a controlled motion.

Repetitions: Begin with 4–10 repetitions, gradually increasing to 15–20 as you build strength.

Mini Squat

Instructions: Stand behind a sturdy chair. Slowly bend your knees, and sit your weight back into your heels, lowering slightly into a mini squat.

For an added challenge, lift your toes slightly to exaggerate the weight in your heels. Keep your spine long and avoid rounding your back. Hold for a few breaths, then rise back to standing.

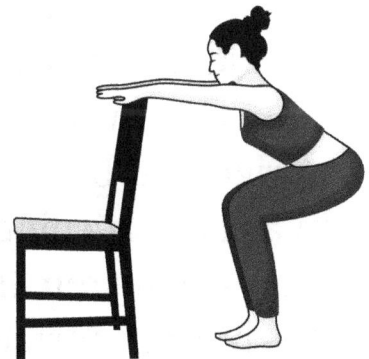

Repetitions: Repeat 3-5 times, holding each squat for several breaths.

Progression Options

Half Squat

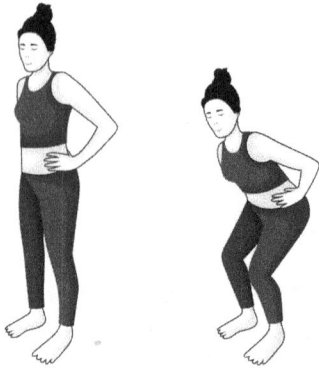

If you feel confident, perform a half squat without holding onto the chair. Keep your hands on your hips or extend them forward for balance.

Repetitions: Begin with 8–10 repetitions, aiming for 2–3 sets.

Full Squats

When you feel strong enough, progress to a full squat

Instructions: Stand with feet shoulder-width apart, slightly turning your toes outward. Keeping your chest upright, sit back and down, as if sitting in a chair, keeping weight in your heels. Stop when your thighs are parallel to the ground or when you reach a comfortable depth.

Push through your heels to rise back up.

Repetitions: Start with 3 sets of 6-8 repetitions. For guidance on depth, place a chair behind you.

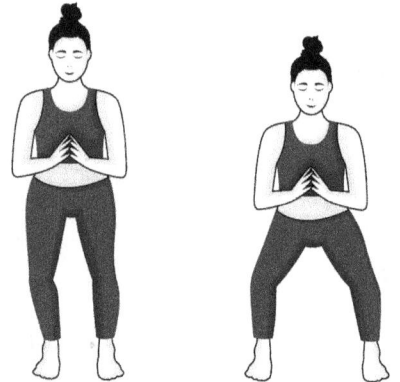

Chair Pose Hovering Above Chair

Instructions: Sit tall in a sturdy chair, feet flat on the ground. Raise your arms above your head, reaching upward. Engage your core, press down through your feet, and rise just an inch or two above the seat, hovering.

Hold for a few breaths, then sit back down with control.

Repetitions: Repeat this hover 3–5 times, focusing on deep breaths and controlled movements.

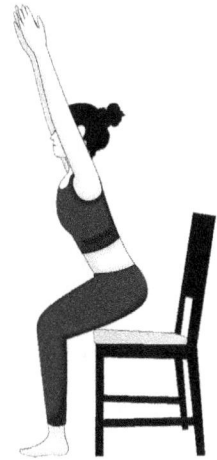

Hamstring Sets

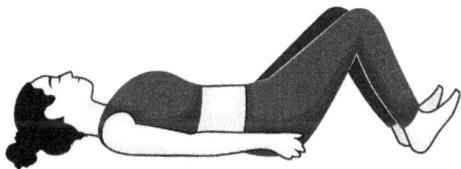

Instructions: Lie on your back with knees bent and feet flat, toes pointing up. Press your heels into the ground, engaging your hamstrings.

Hold the contraction for 6–10 seconds, then release. **Repetitions:** Repeat up to 15-20 times, resting briefly between each repetition.

Straight Leg Raise

Instructions: Lie on your back with your spine flush against the floor, avoiding any arching. Bend one knee with your foot flat on the floor, and keep the other leg straight. Tighten the thigh muscles of your straight leg and pull your toes toward you.

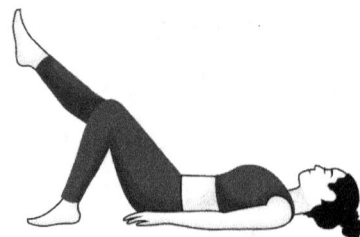

Slowly lift your leg to the height of the bent knee, then lower it back down.

Repetitions: Perform 6-8 repetitions per leg, then switch. Aim for 3 sets.

Bridge

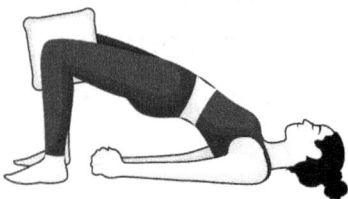

Instructions: Lie on your back with your knees bent, feet flat on the floor, and a comfortable distance from your hips. Squeeze a folded pillow between your knees for added inner thigh activation.

Press through your heels and lift your hips, forming a straight line from shoulders to knees.

Hold briefly, then lower back down.

Repetitions: Repeat 6–8 times, gradually increasing as you build strength.

Knee Extension

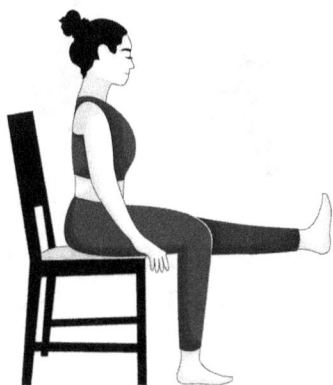

Instructions: Sit upright in a chair with feet flat on the floor.

Extend one leg straight, tightening the thigh muscle and pulling your toes back toward you.

Hold the extended position for 10 seconds, then lower your foot back down.

Repetitions: Perform 8-10 repetitions per leg, then switch. Aim for 3 sets.

Calf Raises

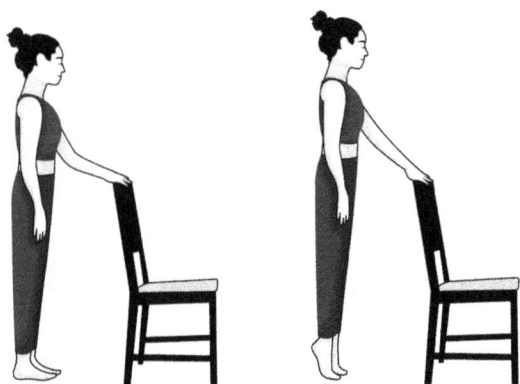

Instructions: Lift your heels as high as comfortable, hold them briefly, then lower them back down.

Repetitions: Complete 8–10 repetitions, gradually working up to 3 sets. For added challenge, try lowering on one foot.

Step-ups

Instructions: Stand in front of a sturdy step or low platform, about 8–10 inches high, or you can use the stairs. Ensure your foot fits comfortably on the step. Place your right foot on the step, then press down to lift yourself onto the step. Keep your body straight, don't lean forward.

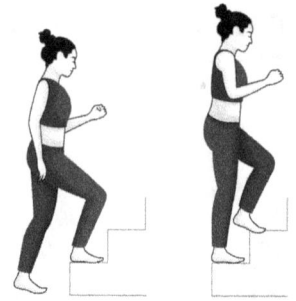

Bring your left foot up to meet the right. Step down with your left foot, followed by the right. Maintain a steady, controlled pace. Make sure that your knees are over your ankle, forming 90-degree angle and that your knees are not caving in.

Repetitions: Perform 8–12 step-ups per leg, working up to 2–3 sets.

Step Downs

Instructions: Stand on a step or platform with one foot, letting the opposite foot hang slightly off the edge. Slowly lower your hanging foot to the ground, keeping control and allowing the knee to bend slightly.

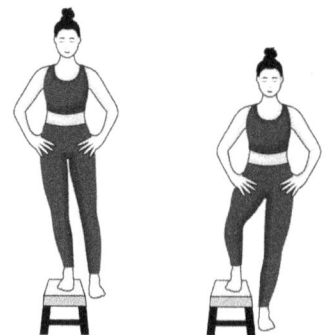

Press back up through your standing leg to return to the starting position.

Repetitions: Complete 6–8 step-downs per leg, aiming for 2–3 sets.

Butt Kicks

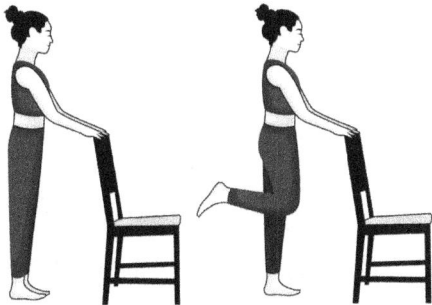

Instructions: Stand tall, holding onto a stable surface if needed.

Bend one knee, lifting your heel toward your glutes, as if trying to kick your but.

Repetitions: Complete up to 10-15 kicks per side, aim for 3 sets.

Single Leg Bridge

Instructions: Lie on your back with your knees bent and feet flat on the floor.

Lift your hips up to form a straight line from shoulders to knees.

Extend one leg straight out, keeping your hips level.

Hold for a few breaths, then lower and switch legs.

Repetitions: Repeat 2–3 times per leg, gradually increasing hold time.

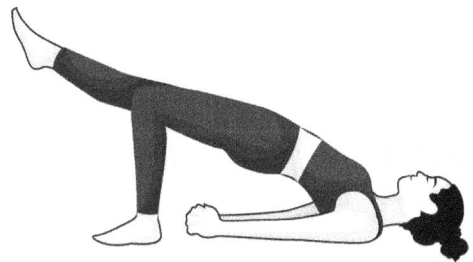

Lunge

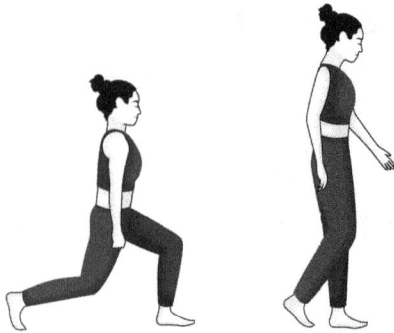

Instructions: Stand upright with feet hip-width apart.

Step back with your right foot, lowering your body until your left knee is aligned with your left ankle.

Keep your torso upright and hold briefly, then push back up to the starting position.

Repeat on the opposite side.

Repetitions: Complete 4–6 lunges per side, gradually increasing repetitions as you build strength.

Side Leg Raises

Instructions: Lie on your side with both legs straight, stacking one leg on top of the other.

Lift the top leg as high as comfortable, keeping your toes pointed forward.

Lower your leg back down slowly, keeping control.

Repetitions: Perform 6-8 raises on each side, aiming for 2–3 sets.

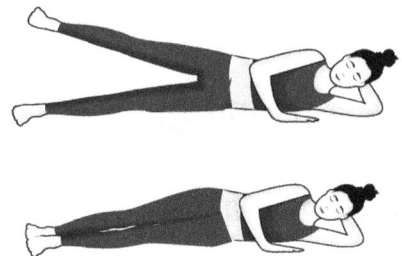

Side Leg Lifts

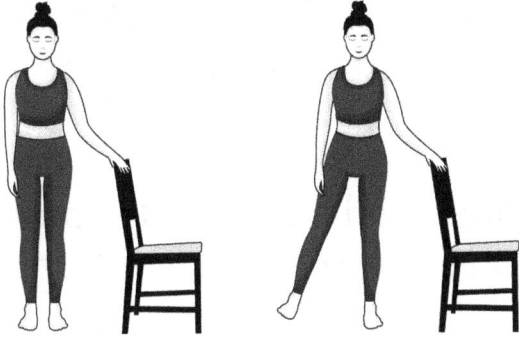

Instructions: Stand beside a chair, holding it for support.

Lift one leg out to the side without leaning or rotating your torso.

Lower your leg back down with control, focusing on smooth movements.

Repetitions: Complete 6–8 lifts per leg, aiming for 2–3 sets.

Front Leg Raise

Instructions: Stand upright with feet hip-width apart.

Lift one leg straight out in front of you, keeping your core engaged and torso stable.

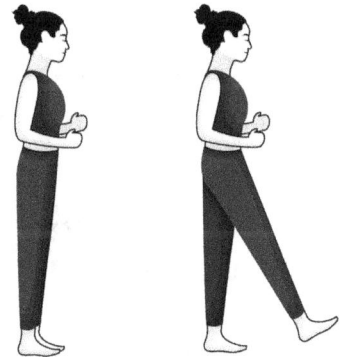

Hold briefly, then lower back to the starting position.

Repetitions: Perform 6–8 lifts per leg, gradually working up to 2–3 sets.

Leg Swings

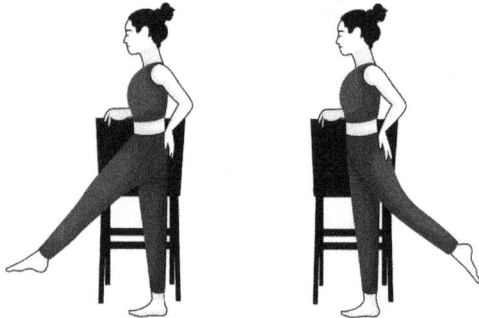

Instructions: Stand beside a chair or wall for balance.

Swing one leg forward and back in a controlled motion, keeping your torso steady.

Focus on smooth, fluid movements.

Repetitions: Complete 8–10 swings per leg, repeating for 2–3 sets.

Hip Extension

Instructions: Stand behind a chair with your hands resting on the back.

Shift your weight onto your right foot, then extend your left leg straight back.

Lift your left leg slightly, hold for a few breaths, then lower it back down.

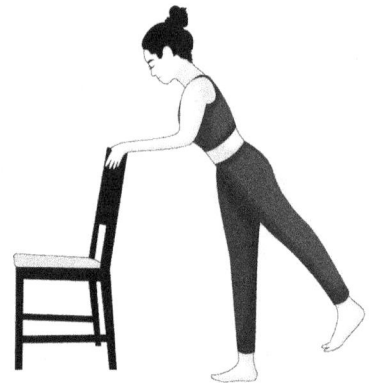

Repetitions: Repeat 8–10 times per leg, aiming for 2–3 sets.

Prone Leg Raises

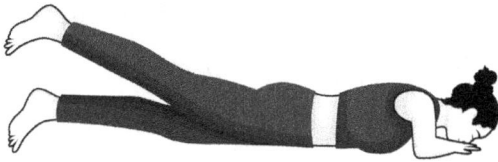

Instructions: Lie face down with your arms resting under your head.

Lift one leg slightly off the floor, keeping it straight.

Hold for a few seconds, then lower with control.

Repetitions: Perform 8–10 raises per leg, gradually increasing as you feel stronger.

Hip Abduction

Instructions: Lie on your right side with your right leg bent at a 45-degree angle. Keep your left leg straight and stacked on top of your bent right leg.

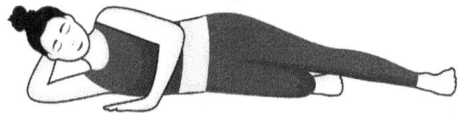

Keep your top leg straight, lifting it to a 45-degree angle without bending or locking your knee.

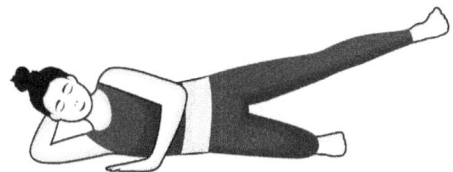

Hold briefly, then slowly lower your leg back to the starting position.

Repetitions: Perform 8–10 repetitions per leg, gradually working up to 3 sets.

Hip Adduction variation

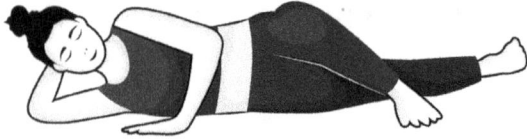

Instructions: Lie on your side. Cross the top leg over the other leg, resting it in front. Lift the straight leg about 6–8 inches off the ground, hold for a few seconds, then lower.

Repetitions: Aim for 8-10 repetitions, completing 2–3 sets per leg.

Monster Walk (Side Steps)

Instructions: Bend your knees slightly and take small side steps to the left and then to the right.

Take 8–10 steps to one side, space-dependent, and then change direction.

Repetitions: Perform 2–3 sets in each direction.

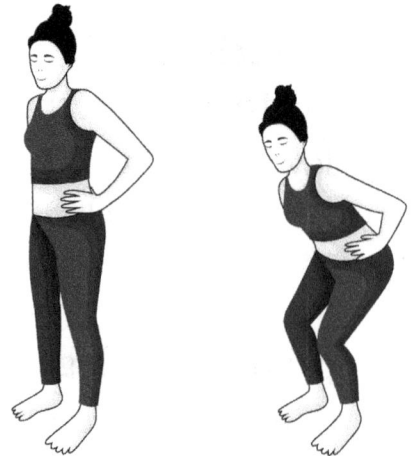

Side Lunge

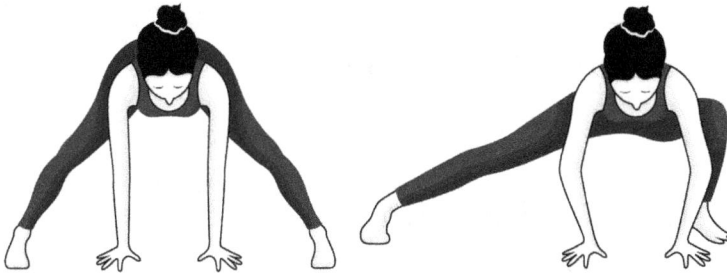

Instructions: Stand upright with feet wider than shoulder-width apart.

Slowly lunge to one side, bending your knee and shifting weight onto the lunging leg.

Keep your opposite leg straight, feeling a stretch in the inner thigh.

Hold briefly, then return to standing and switch sides.

Repetitions: Perform 4–6 lunges per side, working up to 2 sets.

Note: If you feel any pain or discomfort with this exercise, please skip it. Focus on other exercises that feel right for you. It might take some time to build up, or perhaps lunges just aren't the best fit for you right now. Listen to your body and go at your own pace.

Clamshell

Instructions: Lie on your side with your knees bent at a 45-degree angle.

Keeping your feet together, lift your top knee as high as comfortable, without shifting your hips.

Lower your knee back down, focusing on a slow, controlled movement.

Repetitions: Complete 8-10 clamshells per side, working up to 2–3 sets.

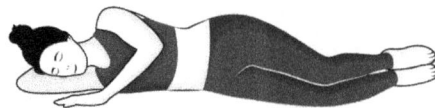

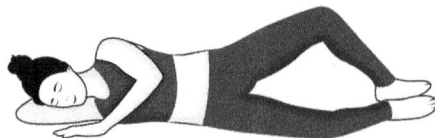

The Importance of Stretching for Knee Health

Strength exercises are essential to support your knee health, but stretching is no less. Strengthening exercises build the muscles around your knees, but stretching keeps those muscles flexible, reducing stiffness and easing movement. When strength and flexibility team up, your knees become better equipped to handle everyday activities.

Why Stretching Matters for Your Knees

Over time, the muscles and tissues around your knees can tighten up, leading to that uncomfortable, "rusty hinge" feeling. Stretching helps ease tension and promotes smoother movement. Here's how it benefits knee health:

- **Increases Flexibility and Range of Motion:** Flexible muscles around the knee—like the quadriceps, hamstrings, and calves—enable the knee joint to move more freely. This increased range of motion makes bending, extending, and rotating the knee easier. For example, flexible hamstrings reduce knee strain when sitting or going downstairs.

Reduces Muscle Tension: Tight muscles can pull on the knee joint and cause discomfort. Regular stretching releases this tension, making the muscles around the knee more relaxed and less likely to disrupt joint alignment. This is especially important for the quadriceps and calves, which can create additional stress on the knee when overly tight.

Increases Circulation: Stretching boosts muscle blood flow, delivering oxygen and nutrients that aid in recovery and repair. Improved circulation helps reduce inflammation and stiffness, making movement more comfortable. Healthy blood flow also supports cartilage health, which cushions the knee joint.

Addressing Muscle Imbalances: Knee pain often stems from muscle imbalances around the joint. Tight or overactive muscles like the quadriceps or hamstrings can pull unevenly on the knee, causing discomfort. Stretching lengthens these muscles. It reduces the pull on the knee joint and promotes balanced support from surrounding muscles. This helps align the knee properly and reduces strain.

Helps with Knee Joint Alignment: Stiff muscles around the knee can lead to poor alignment and increased joint strain. Flexible quadriceps and hamstrings contribute to balanced movement. It reduces the risk of misalignment and pain. Stretching supports proper knee positioning, which is essential for stability and comfort during daily activities.

🌿 **Supports a Better Range of Motion:** Stretching enhances range of motion, making it easier to perform daily activities without discomfort. When flexibility is better, the knee can move fully and without restriction, which is particularly beneficial for tasks involving bending, squatting, or extending the leg.

🌿 **Supports Balance and Reduces Injury Risk:** Flexible muscles improve balance, helping to prevent falls and knee injuries. Stretching keeps muscles responsive, enabling the knee to adapt better to sudden movements or changes in position.

Stretching Exercises for Healthy Knees

Half-Kneeling Hip Flexor Stretch

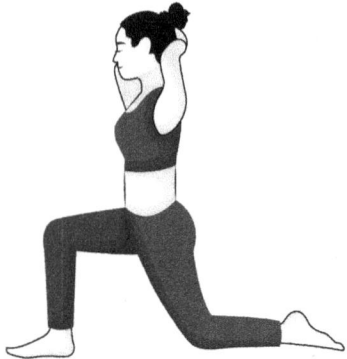

Instructions: Start in a kneeling position on the floor. For added comfort, place an exercise mat or towel under your knee.

Step your right foot forward, creating a 90-degree angle with your right knee, while extending your left leg straight behind you with the top of the foot resting on the floor.

Place your hands on your hips or behind your head. Engage your glutes to gently tuck your pelvis under, creating a stable and aligned base. Keeping your back straight and gaze forward, slowly shift your weight forward until you feel a stretch along the front of your right hip.

Hold the position for 2 to 3 breaths, breathing deeply and avoiding any bouncing or sudden movements.

To finish, shift your weight back, return your left knee to the floor, and switch to the other side.

Benefits: This stretch is especially helpful for those who sit for long periods, as it releases tight hip flexors, which can relieve knee strain and improve posture.

Supine Hamstring Floor Stretch

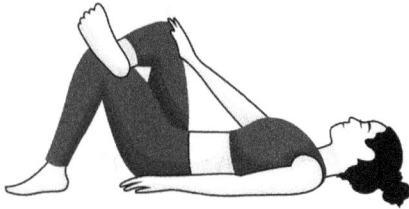

Instructions: Bend both knees, keeping your feet flat on the mat and hip-width apart. Lift your right knee towards your chest and cross the right ankle over your left knee.

Repetitions: Hold the stretch for 20–30 seconds, or 2 – 3 breaths, performing 2–3 sets per leg.

Standing Calf Stretch

Instructions: Stand facing a wall, placing your hands on it for support.

Step one foot back, keeping the heel flat and toes forward.

Bend your front knee slightly and press your back heel down to feel a stretch in the calf.

Hold briefly, then switch legs.

Repetitions: Hold each stretch for 20–30 seconds, or 2 – 3 breaths, repeating 2–3 times per leg.

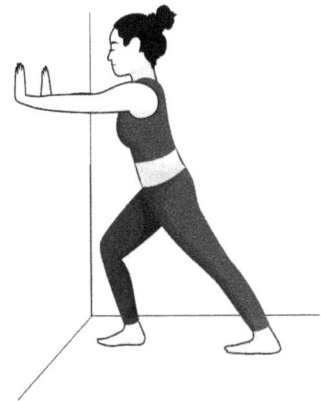

Hamstrings Stretch Lying

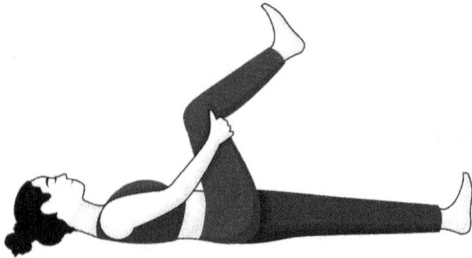

Instructions: Lie on the floor with both legs straightened.

Lift one leg off of the floor and bring the knee toward your chest. Clasp your hands behind your thigh below your knee. If you can't reach, use the strap or the towel, wrapping it behind the thigh. Use the strap to gently pull your leg toward you, keeping your opposite leg straight. If it's too much, bend the opposite leg for support.

Hold the stretch, then lower and repeat with the other leg.

Repetitions: Hold each stretch for 20–30 seconds, or 2 – 3 breaths. Repeat 2–3 times per leg.

Do not put your hands at your knee joint and pull.

If you feel ready, ease into a deeper stretch.

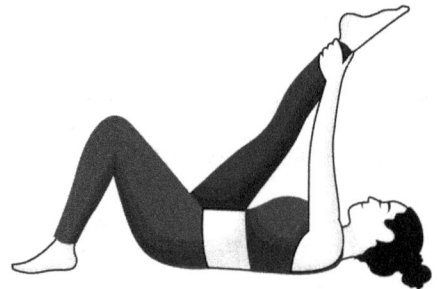

Quadriceps Stretch

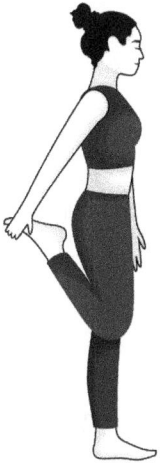

Instructions: Stand beside a sturdy chair or wall for balance.

Bend one knee, bringing your heel toward your glutes, and hold your ankle with your hand.

Keep your knees close together, gently pulling your heel until you feel a stretch along your thigh. Hold briefly, then switch legs.

Repetitions: Hold each stretch for 20–30 seconds, or 2–3 breaths, repeating 2–3 times per leg.

Seated Quad Stretch

Instructions: Sit on the edge of a chair with one foot flat and the other leg extended behind you.

Keep your torso upright, gently leaning back to feel a stretch in your thigh.

Hold the position, then switch legs.

Repetitions: Hold each stretch for 20–30 seconds per leg, performing 2–3 times.

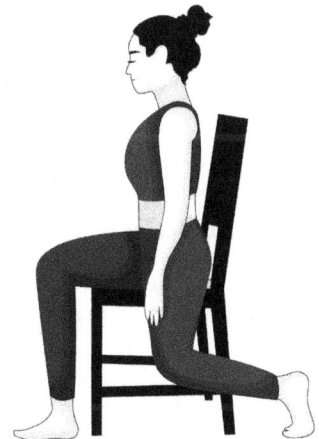

Prone Quad Stretch

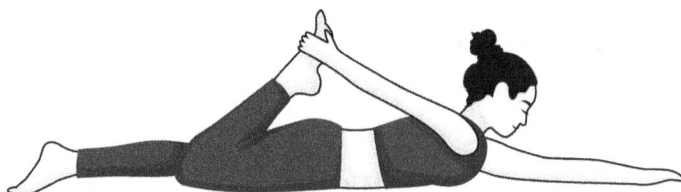

Instructions: Lie face down on the floor with your legs extended and arms at your sides or in front of you.

Bend your right knee and reach back with your right hand to grab your right ankle, just above your foot.

Gently pull your foot and shin toward your glutes until you feel a moderate stretch in the front of your right thigh.

If it's difficult to reach your ankle, use a strap, belt, or towel wrapped around your right foot. Hold the strap with both hands, pulling it over your left shoulder to bring your right heel toward your glute.

Keep your knees close together, and avoid lifting your hip off the ground.

Hold for 20–30 seconds, breathing deeply, then release and switch legs.

Repetitions: Repeat 2–3 times per leg, focusing on a slow and controlled stretch.

Seated Figure Four

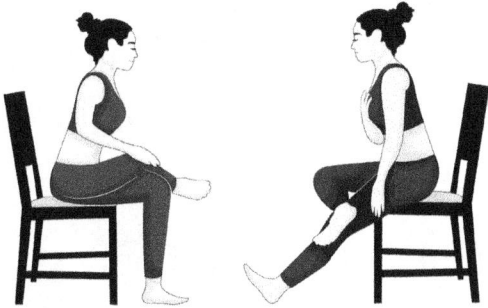

Instructions: Sit on a chair with your back straight and feet flat on the floor.

Place your right ankle on top of your left knee. Or if it's too difficult, straighten the left leg.

Keeping your back straight, gently lean forward from your hips until you feel a stretch in your right hip and outer thigh.

Repetitions: Perform 2–3 stretches on each side. Hold the stretch for 20-30 seconds.

One Knee Stretch

Instructions: Sit upright in a chair with feet flat on the ground.

Pull your right knee toward your chest, using your hands to gently press your thigh toward you.

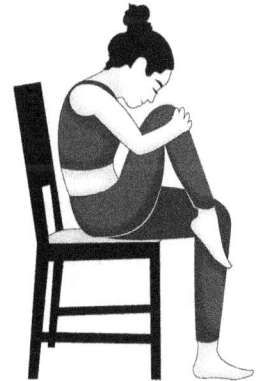

Flex your head slightly forward to bring your face toward your knee, feeling a stretch along your back and hamstring.

Repetitions: Repeat 2–3 times on each side. Hold the stretch for 10-15 seconds.

Hamstring Stretch

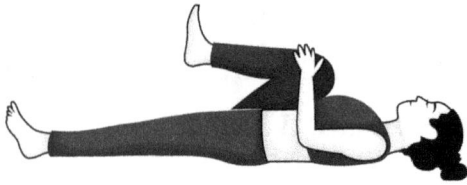

Instructions: Lie down on your back on a comfortable surface. Extend your right leg straight out in front of you.

Bend your left knee, keeping your foot flat on the floor.

Wrap your hands around the back of your left thigh or gently hold just above your knee.

Slowly pull your left leg toward you until you feel a comfortable stretch along the back of your thigh.

Repetitions: Hold the stretch for each leg for 20 seconds, breathing deeply. Repeat a few times.

Hamstring Stretch

Instructions: Sit near the edge of a chair with your right leg extended straight out, and toes pointing up.

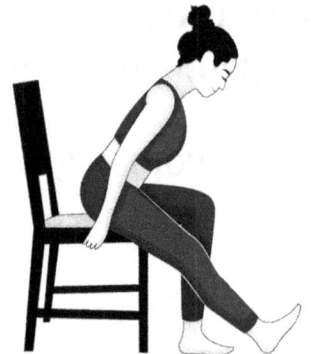

Lean forward gently from your hips until you feel a stretch along the back of your extended leg. Keep your back straight and avoid bouncing.

Hold for 20–30 seconds, breathing deeply, then switch legs.

Repetitions: Perform 2–3 times per leg.

About Crossover Standing Forward Bend

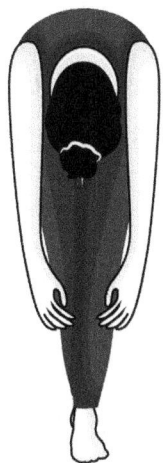

Instructions: Stand upright and cross your right foot in front of your left.

Slowly bend forward from your hips, reaching your hands toward the floor.

Keep your knees slightly bent and let your upper body relax into the stretch.

Hold for 20–30 seconds, then return to standing and switch legs.

Repetitions: Repeat 2–3 times on each side.

Standing Hip Crossover Stretch

Instructions: Stand beside a wall for support, crossing your right leg behind your left.

Shift your hips toward the wall, feeling a stretch along the outer hip and thigh.

Hold for 20–30 seconds, breathing deeply, then switch sides.

Repetitions: Perform 2–3 times per side.

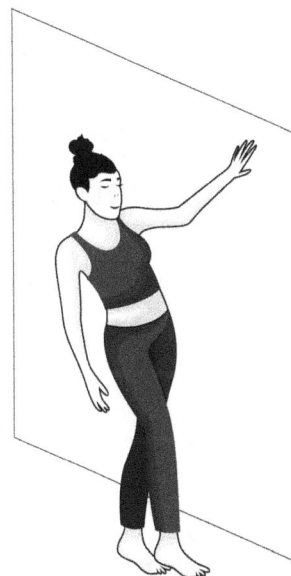

Adductor Stretch

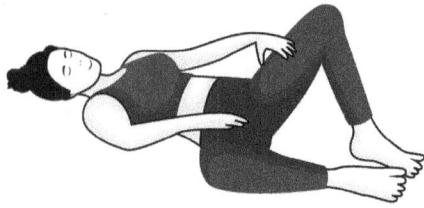

Instructions: Lie on your back and bend your both knees. Lower your knees outward to the sides while keeping both feet together.

Use your hand to gently press on the inner thigh if needed, feeling a stretch in the adductor muscles.

Hold for 20–30 seconds, then bring the knee back to the center and switch sides.

Repetitions: Repeat 2–3 times on each side.

Seated Forward Bend Pose Chair against Wall

Instructions: Sit on the edge of a chair with legs extended forward.

Inhale as you raise your arms, and exhale as you fold forward from the hips.

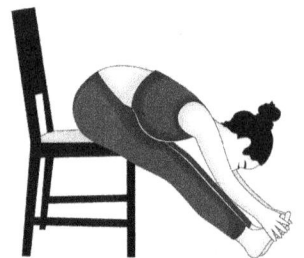

Hold for 2-5 breaths, keeping the spine elongated.

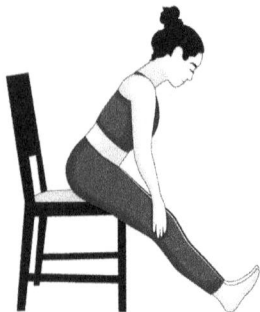

Repetitions: Perform 2–3 times, taking breaths to relax between stretches.

If you cannot reach your toes, then place your arms above the knees.

Knee Strengthening Routines

Day 1

Knee Extension

Standing Hamstring Curls

Repeat 15-20 times each leg, then switch

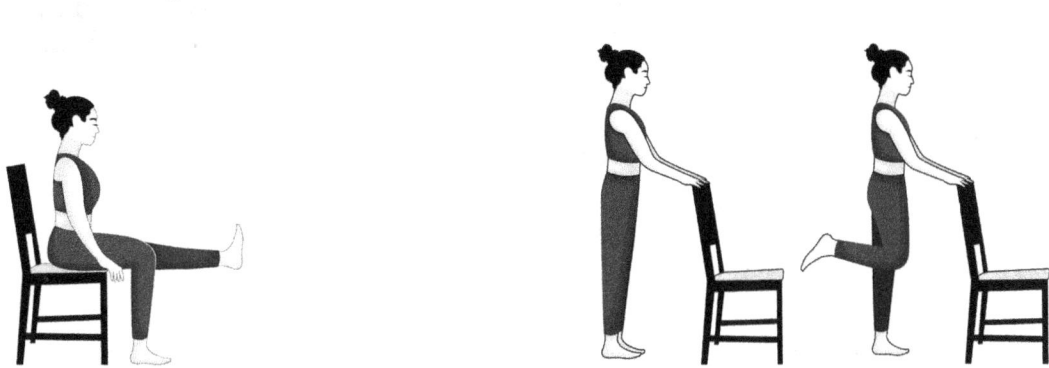

Sit to Stand

Repeat 15-20 times

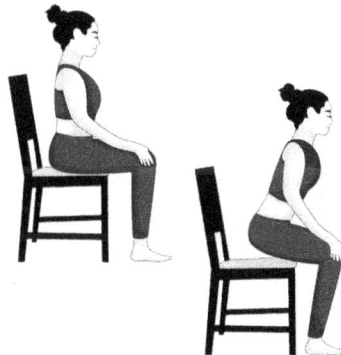

Repeat the routine 2-3 times.

Day 2

Side Leg Lifts

Repeat 10-15 per side

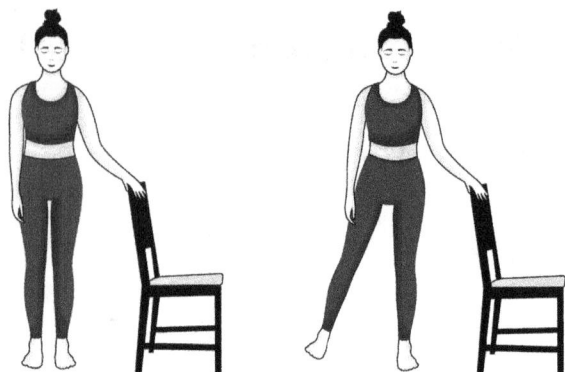

Sit to Stand

Repeat 15-20 times

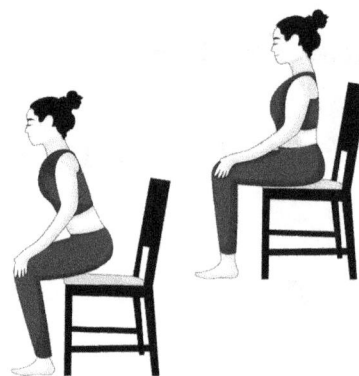

Butt Kicks

Repeat 10-15 per leg

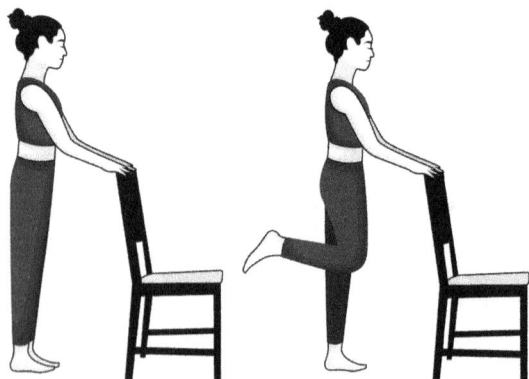

Clamshell

Repeat 8-10 times

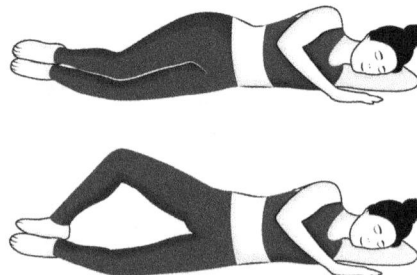

Prone Quad Stretch

Hold 2-3 breaths per leg

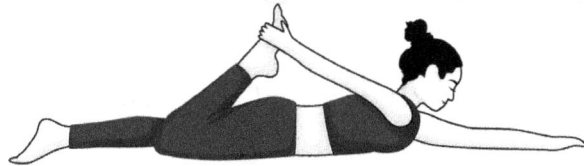

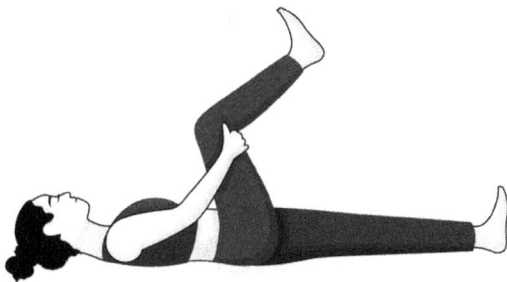

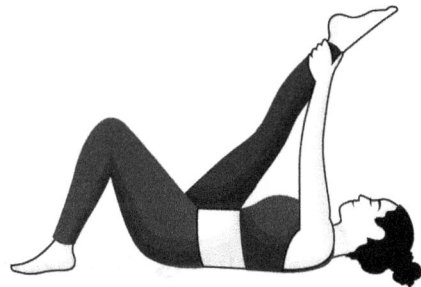

Hamstrings Stretch

Hold 2-3 breaths per leg

Repeat the routine one more time.

Day 3

Standing Calf and Quadriceps Stretch

Hold each leg for 2-3 breaths

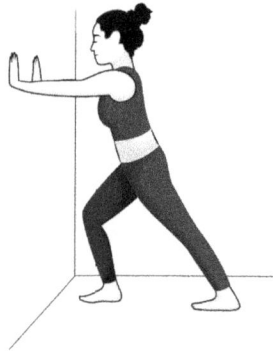

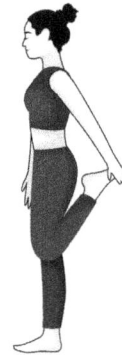

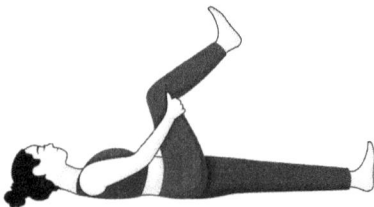

Repeat 2-3 sets

Hamstrings Stretch

Hold each leg for 2-3 breaths

Repeat 2 – 4 sets

Half Squat

Repeat 8-10 times

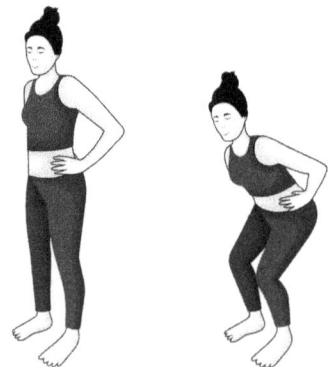

Sets 2-3

Day 4

Standing Hamstring Curls

10-15 each leg, then switch

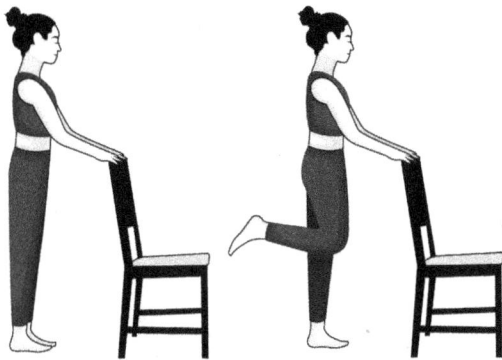

Calf Raises

Repeat 8-10 times

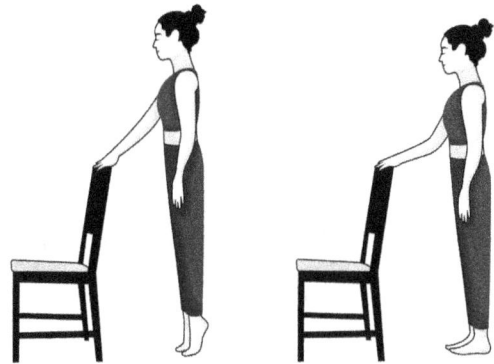

Sets 1-2

Knee Extensions

Straight Leg Raises

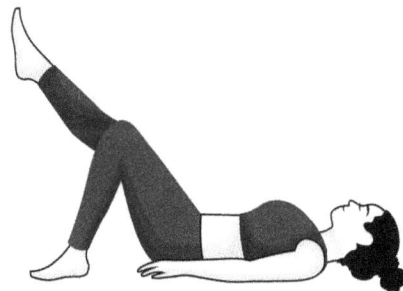

Repeat 10-12 each leg

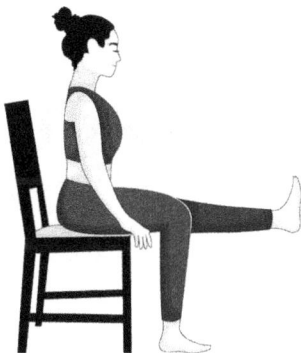

Sets 2-4

Day 5

Prone Hamstring Curl

15-20 each leg

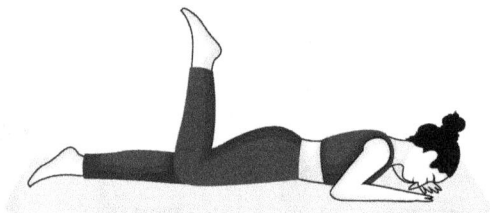

Hip Abduction

Repeat 8-12 per leg

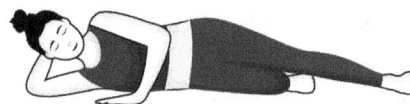

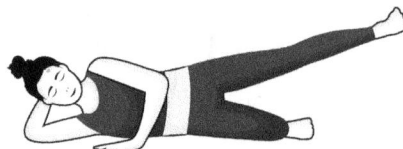

Single Leg Quad and Hamstring Set

Repeat 10-15 each leg

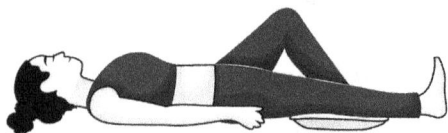

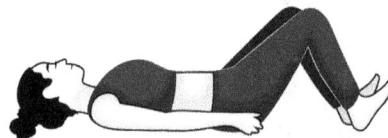

Repeat the entire sequence 2 – 3 times

Day 6

Half Squat

Repeat 8-10

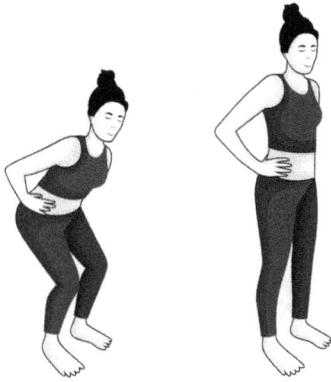

One Leg Backlit

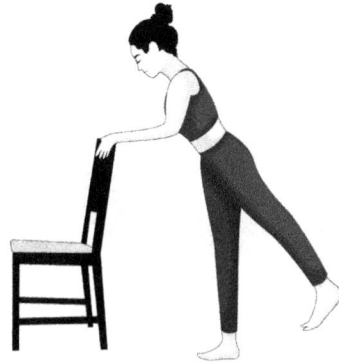

Wall Slides

Repeat 4-10, hold 15-30s

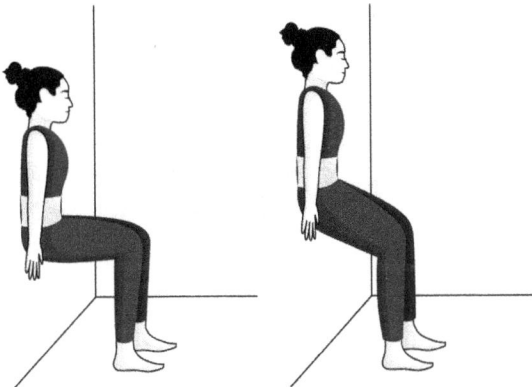

Lunge

Repeat 4-6 one leg

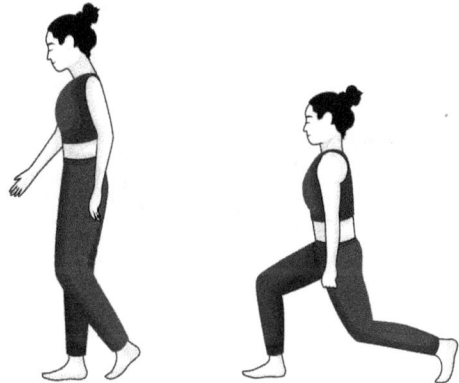

Repeat the routine one more time.

Day 7

Straight Leg Raise

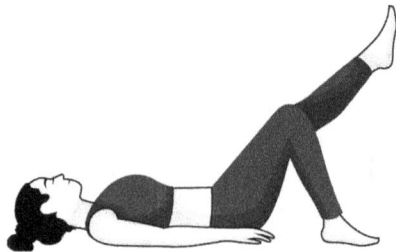

Side Leg Raises

Repeat 6-10 per leg for each exercise

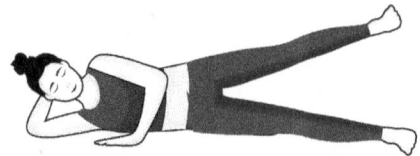

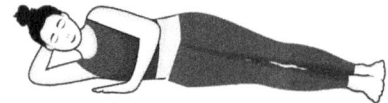

Sets 2-3

Hip Adduction

Prone Hamstring Curl

Repeat 6-10 per leg,
then switch

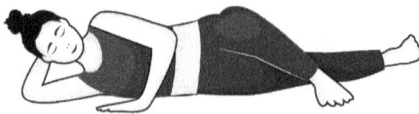

Repeat 10-15 each leg

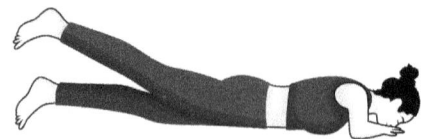

Sets 2-3

Repeat the routine one more time.

Day 8

Supine Hamstring Floor Stretch

Keep the stretch 1-2 breaths each leg

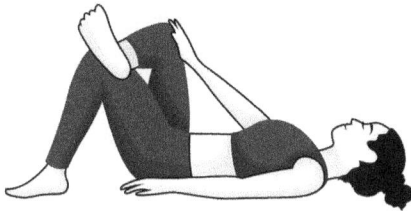

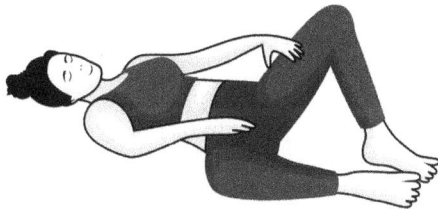

Sets 2-3

Hamstrings Stretch Lying

Hold 30s, Sets 2-3

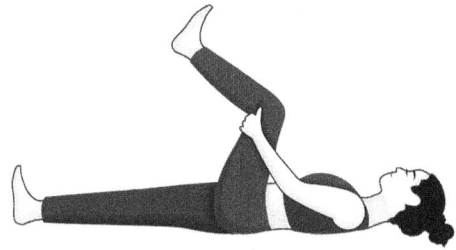

Adductor Stretch Lying

Keep the stretch 1-2 breaths each leg

Sets 2-3

Each Side 2-3 breaths

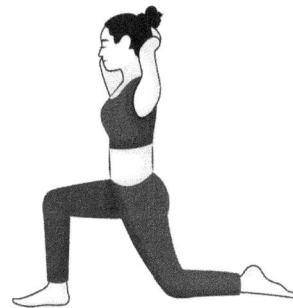

Sets 1

Day 9

Single Leg Quad Sets

Hamstring Sets

Repeat 10-15 each leg

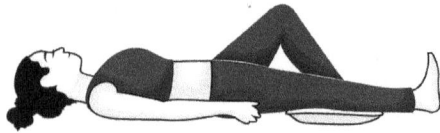

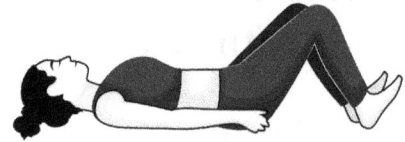

Sets 2-3 each exercise

Straight Leg Raise

Prone Hamstring

Repeat 15-20 each leg

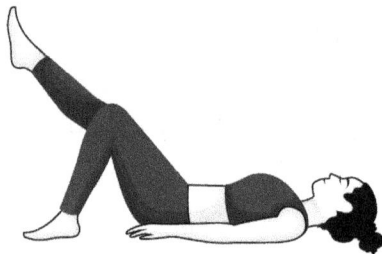

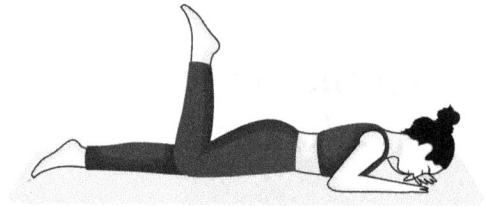

Sets 2-3

Day 10

Wall Slides

Hold 20-30s, repeat 4-10

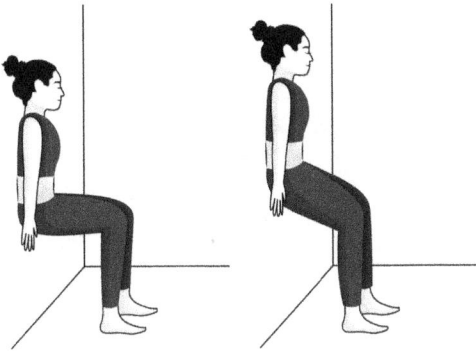

Step-ups

8–12 step-ups per leg

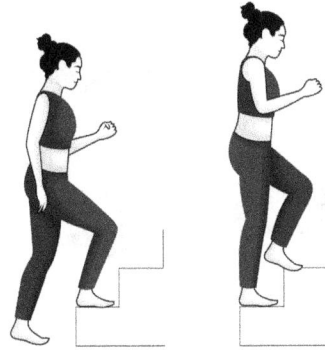

Step Downs

Repeat 8–12 step-downs per leg

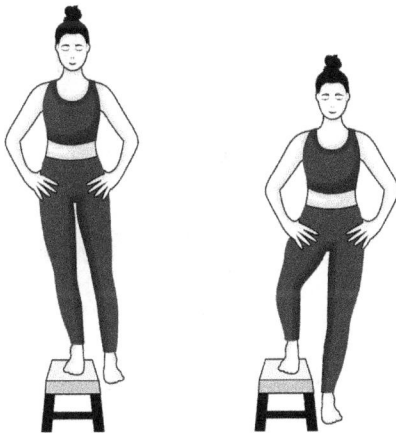

Seated Figure

Hold stretch for 20-30s

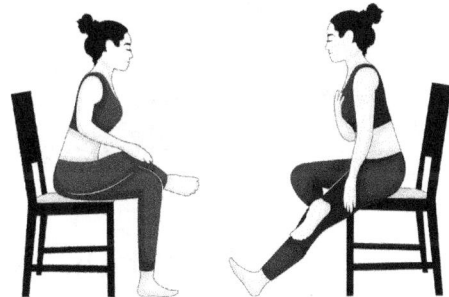

Repeat the entire sequence twice.

Day 11

Clamshell

Bridge

Repeat 8-10 per side, each exercise

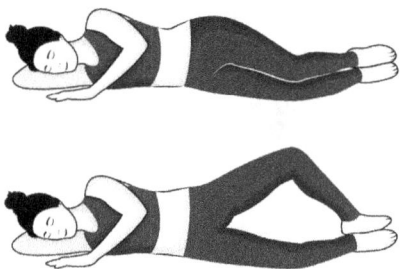

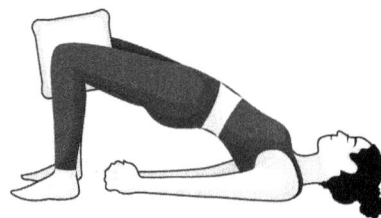

Side Leg Raises

Seated Quad Stretch

Repeat 8-12 per side

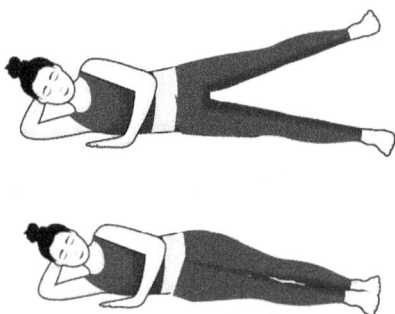

Hold stretch for 20-30s

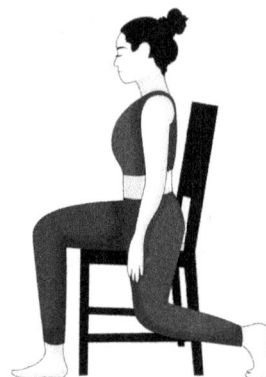

Repeat the entire sequence 2 − 3 times

Day 12

Straight Leg Raise

Side Leg Raises

Repeat 6-8 each leg

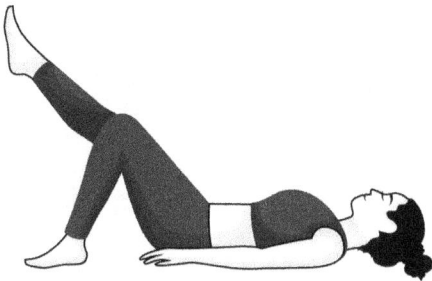

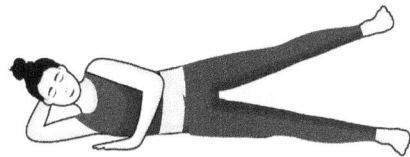

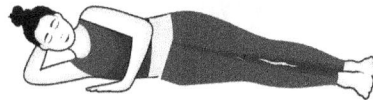

Prone Leg Raises

Repeat 8-10 each leg

Prone Quad Stretch

Hold for 20-30s each leg.

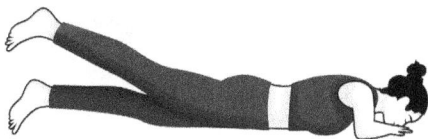

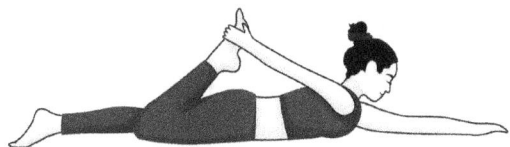

Repeat the entire sequence 2 – 3 times.

Day 13

Lunge

Repeat 4-6 per side

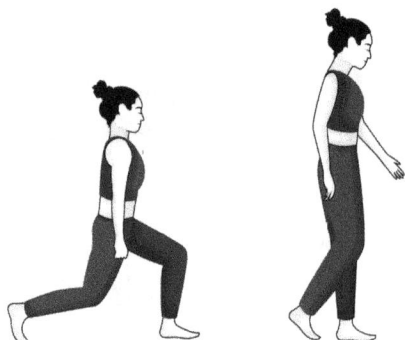

Leg Swings

8-10 per leg

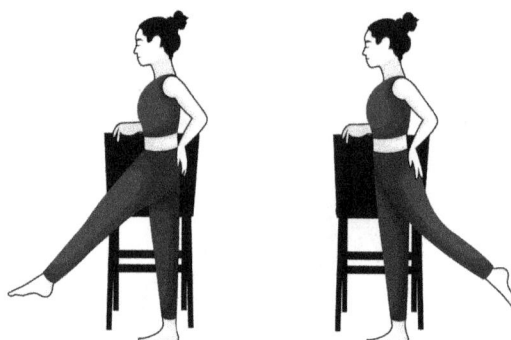

Front Leg Raise

Repeat 6-8 per leg

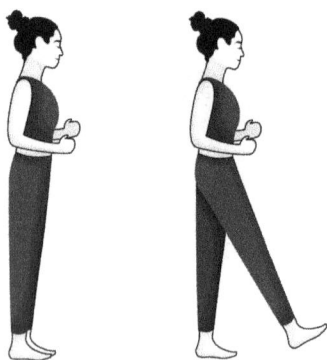

Calf Raises

Repeat 12-14

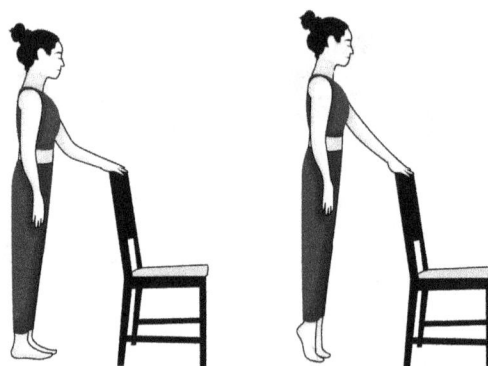

Repeat the entire sequence 2–3 times.

Day 14

Chair Squat

Repeat 8-10

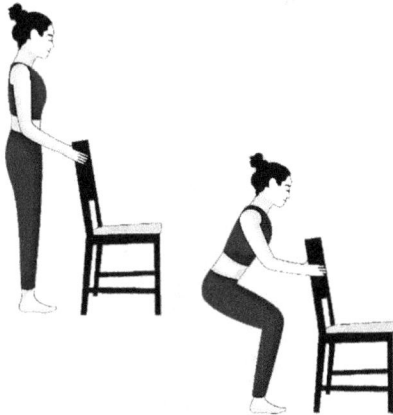

Chair Pose Hovering Above Chair

Hold 20–30s, repeat 2-4

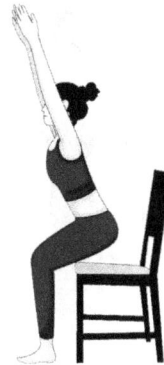

Knee Extension

Repeat 8 – 12 each leg

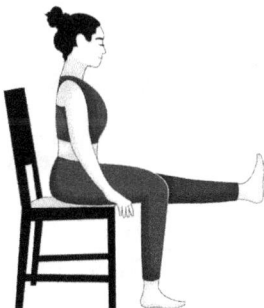

Step-ups

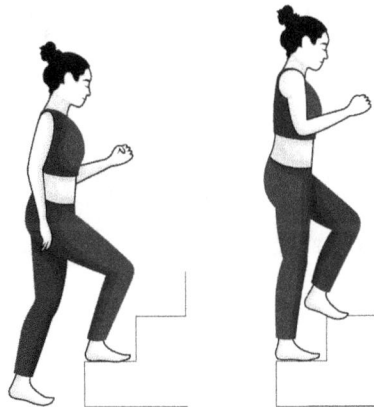

Day 15

Quadriceps Stretch

Kneeling Hip Flexor Stretch

Hold each leg for 2-3 breaths

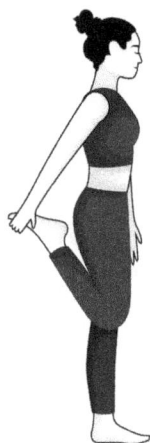

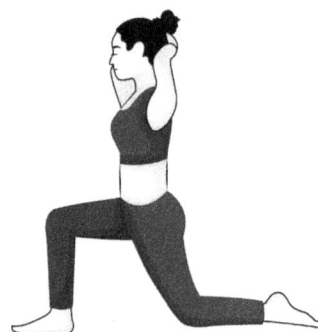

Hamstring and Adductor Stretch Lying

Each leg 1-2 breaths

Hold 2-3 breaths

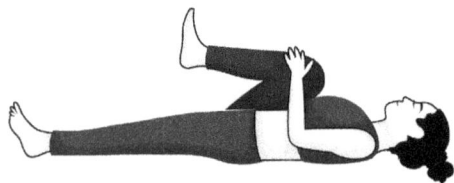

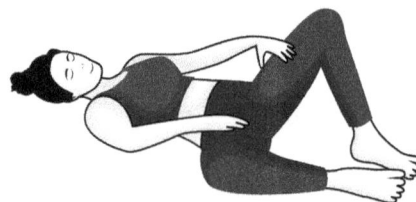

Repeat the entire sequence 2-3 times.

Day 16

One Knee and Hamstring Stretch

Hold for 2-3 breaths

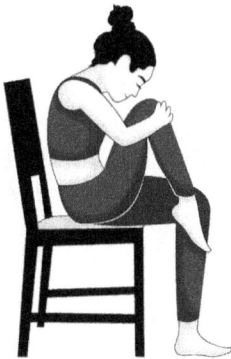

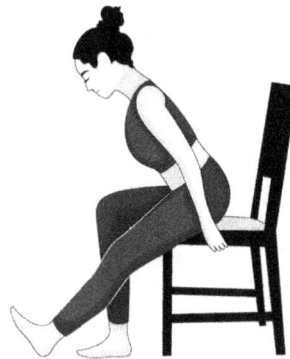

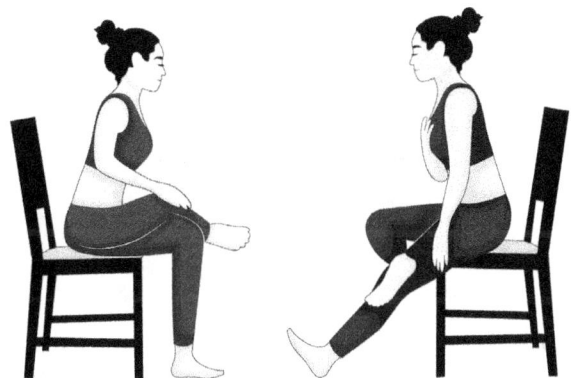

Crossover Standing Forward Bend

Hold for 1-2 breaths

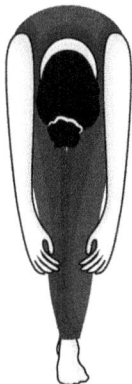

Seated Figure Four

Hold for 2-3 breaths

Repeat the sequence twice.

Day 17

Side Lunge

Repeat 4-6, alternate sides

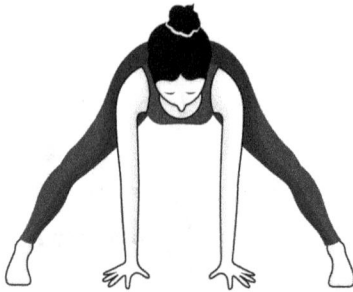

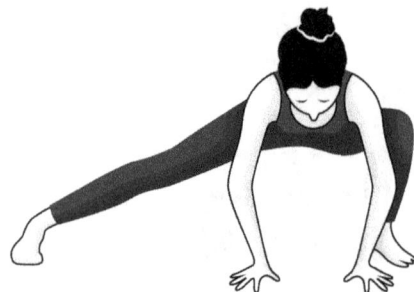

Monster Walk (Side Steps)

Repeat 8-10 one then switch

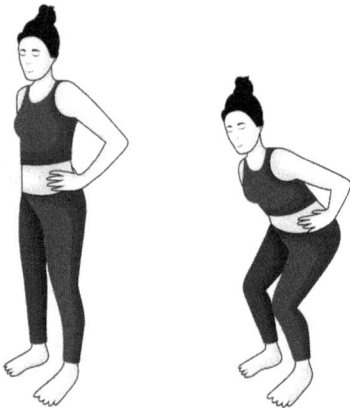

Butt Kicks

Repeat 10-15 per leg

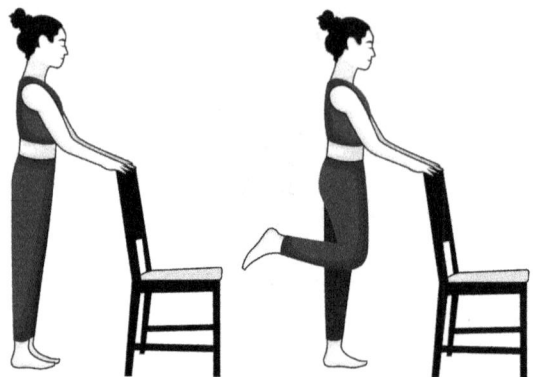

Repeat the sequence 2–3 times.

Hip Adduction variation

Repeat 8-10 times per leg, then switch

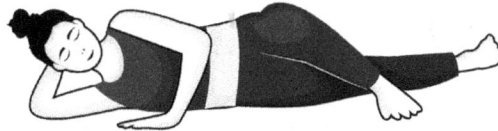

Prone Leg Raises

Repeat 8-10 per leg

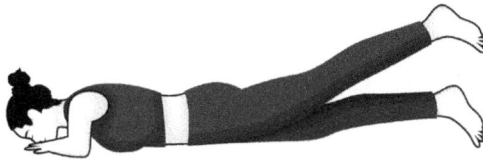

Supine Hamstring Floor Stretch

Hold each leg for 2-3 breaths, repeat 1-2 times

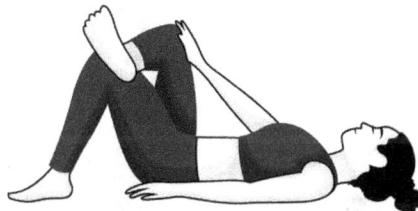

You can repeat the entire sequence 2-3 times.

Day 18

Half-Kneeling Hip Flexor Stretch

Hold each leg for 2-3 breaths, repeat 1-2 times

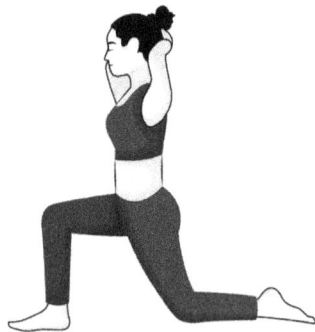

One Leg Opposite Arm Lift

Alternate, 14-16 times

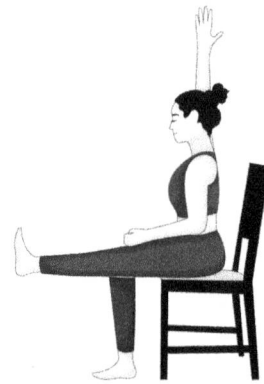

Standing Hamstring Curls

10-15 each leg then switch

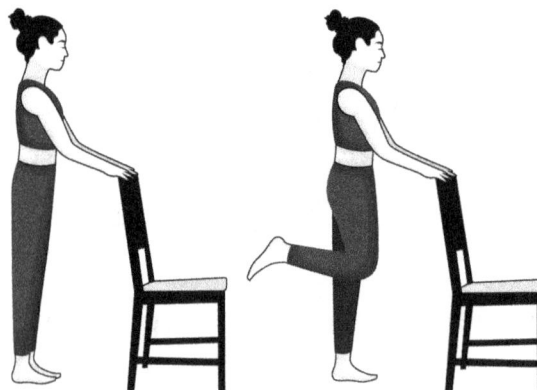

Wall Slides

Hold 20-30s, repeat 4-10

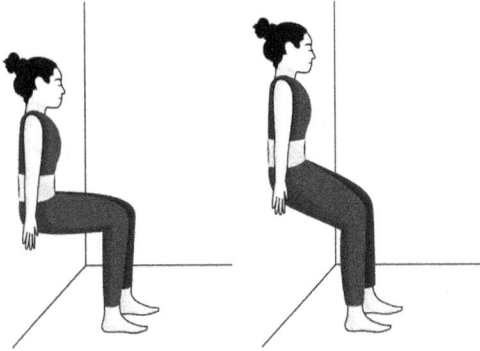

Step-ups

8–12 step-ups per leg

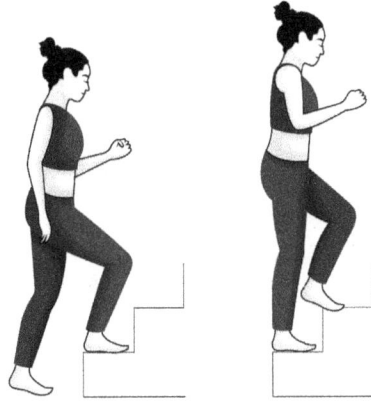

Side Leg Lifts

Repeat each leg 8-12 then switch

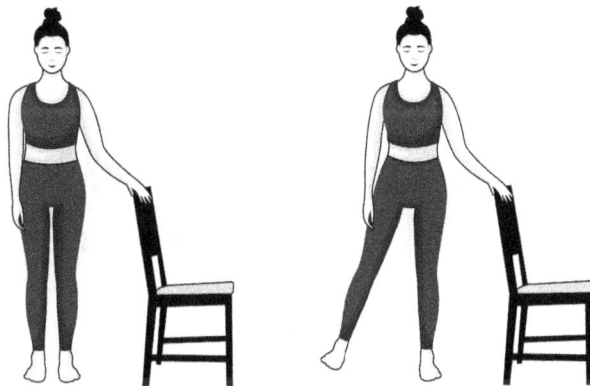

Repeat the sequence twice.

Day 19

Front Leg Raise

Repeat 8-12 per leg, 3 sets

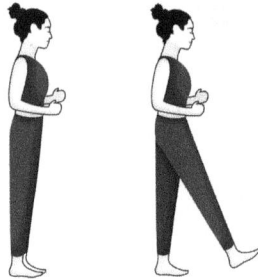

Hip Extension

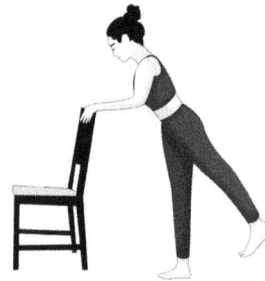

Calf Raises

Repeat 8-12 times   3 sets

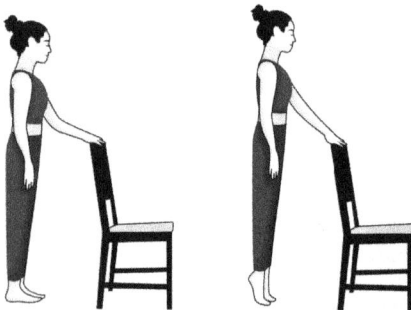

Butt Kicks

10-15 per leg

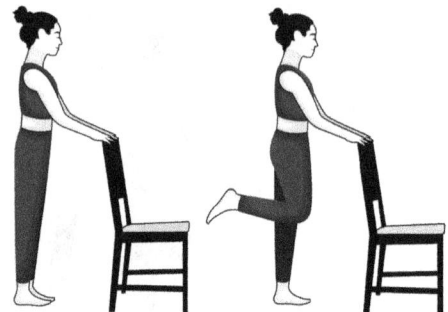

Single Leg Bridge

Hold 2 – 3 breaths,
3 sets each leg.

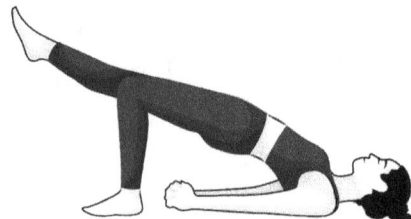

Day 20

Side Leg Raise

Clamshell

Repeat 8-10 per side

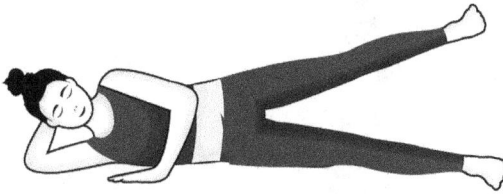

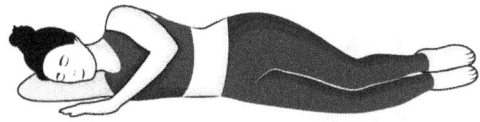

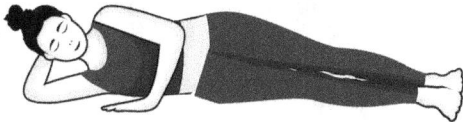

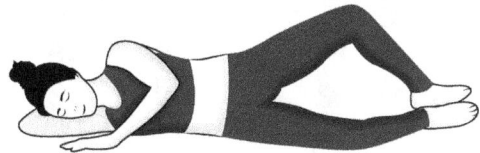

Bridge

Hamstring Sets

Repeat 6-8 times

Repeat 15-20 times

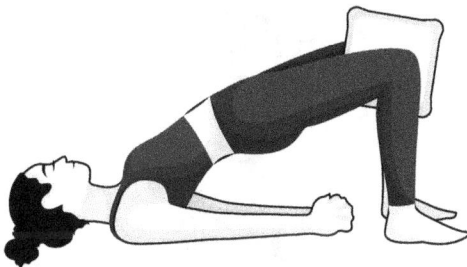

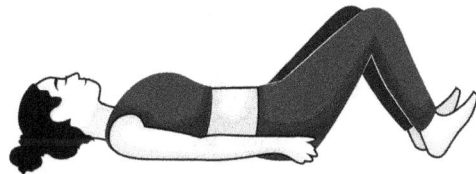

Repeat the entire sequence 2-3 times.

Day 21

Squats

Step-downs

Repeat 6-8 times

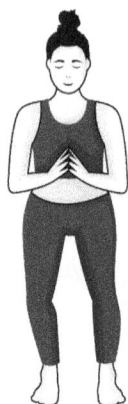

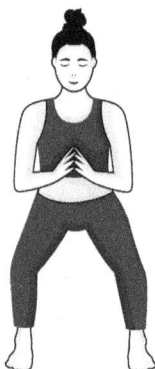

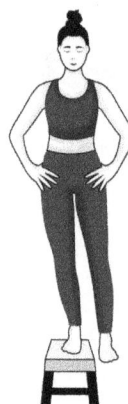

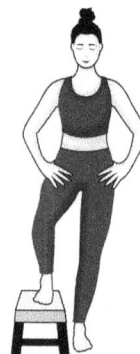

Quadriceps Stretch

Standing Calf Stretch

Hold each leg for 2-3 breaths

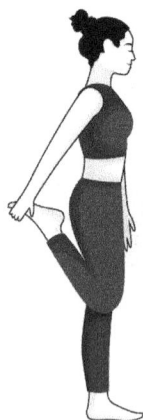

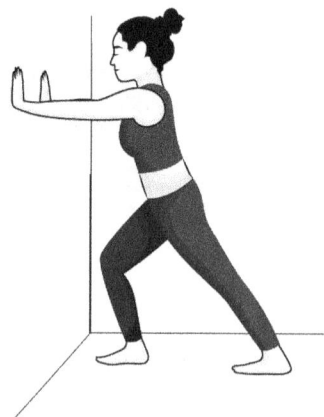

Repeat the entire sequence 2-3 times.

Day 22

Hold each leg for 2-3 breaths.

Supine Hamstring Floor Stretch

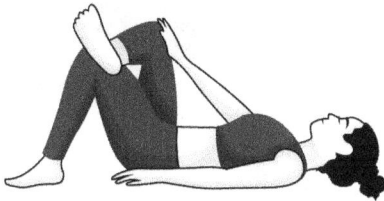

Hamstrings Stretch

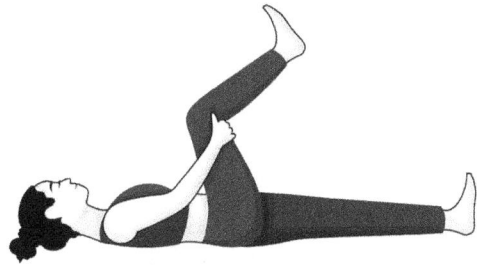

Prone Quad Stretch

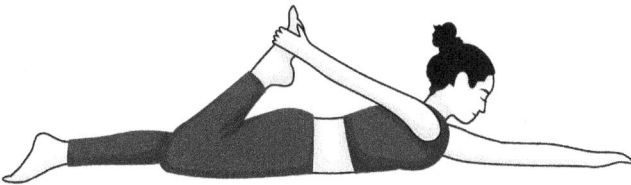

Adductor Stretch

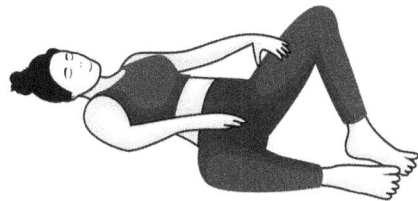

Repeat the sequence twice.

Day 23

Straight Leg Raise

Side Leg Raises

Repeat 6-8 each leg

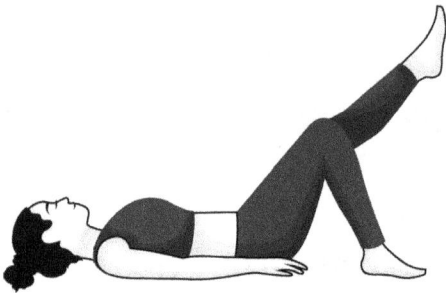

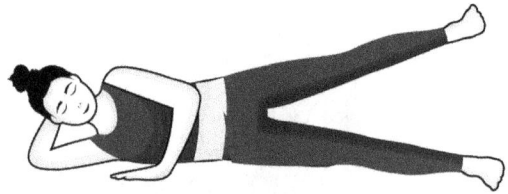

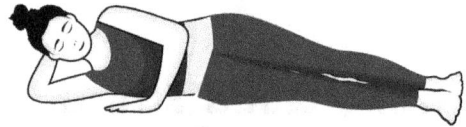

Single Leg Quad and Hamstring Set

Repeat 10-15 each leg

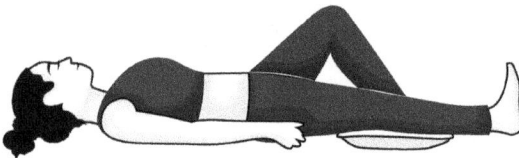

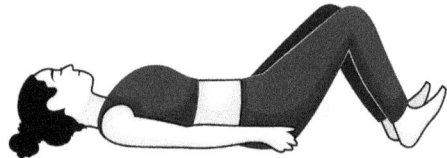

Sets 2-3 each exercise

Repeat the entire sequence 2 – 3 times.

Conclusion

It is not the mountain we conquer, but ourselves.

– Sir Edmund Hillary

Progress doesn't happen overnight, but every little bit counts. Whether it's a few minutes of stretching or completing a full routine, every effort you make is moving you closer to stronger, healthier knees. Some days will feel easier than others, and that's perfectly okay. What matters most is that you keep showing up for yourself.

As you stick with these exercises, you'll start to notice changes—not just in how your knees feel, but in how much more you can do. Everyday activities like climbing stairs, taking a walk, or even chasing after the grandkids will begin to feel easier and more enjoyable.

Remember, every small step you take brings you closer to a more active and confident life. Keep going—you're doing something truly wonderful for yourself!

You Could Be Key to Someone Else's Yoga Journey

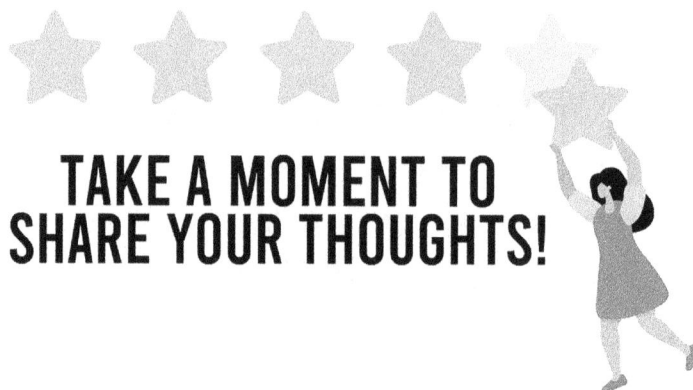

TAKE A MOMENT TO SHARE YOUR THOUGHTS!

Thank you so much for your support. Everyone deserves to access the transformative benefits of well-being, regardless of their physical limitations. With your help, I can ensure this message reaches even more people who need it. By visiting Ottie's Oz's Author Page, you're not just discovering resources—you're joining a movement dedicated to enhancing well-being for all. Explore the page to learn more and help us extend the reach of these essential insights. Thank you for being a part of this vital journey!

References

Here's the reference list in APA style format:

- Articular Cartilage Restoration - OrthoInfo - AAOS. (n.d.). Www.orthoinfo.org. https://orthoinfo.aaos.org/en/treatment/articular-cartilage-restoration

- Nancy Garrick, D. D. (2017, April 7). Reactive Arthritis. National Institute of Arthritis and Musculoskeletal and Skin Diseases. https://www.niams.nih.gov/health-topics/reactive-arthritis/diagnosis-treatment-and-steps-to-take

- Exercise interventions for older adults: A systematic review of meta-analyses. (2020). Journal of Sport and Health Science, 10(1). https://doi.org/10.1016/j.jshs.2020.06.003

- American Psychological Association. (2020, March 4). Working out boosts brain health. American Psychological Association. https://www.apa.org/topics/exercise-fitness/stress

- Arthritis Foundation. (2020). Benefits of Exercise for Osteoarthritis. Arthritis.org. https://www.arthritis.org/health-wellness/healthy-living/physical-activity/getting-started/benefits-of-exercise-for-osteoarthritis

- CDC. (2024, May 7). Physical Activity for Older Adults: An Overview. Physical Activity Basics. https://www.cdc.gov/physical-activity-basics/guidelines/older-adults.html

- Cleveland Clinic. (2018, December 4). Chiropractic Adjustment: What is it, Treatment, Benefits. Cleveland Clinic. https://my.clevelandclinic.org/health/treatments/21033-chiropractic-adjustment

- Corliss, J. (2021, November 1). Cycling: A low-impact exercise that helps the heart. Harvard Health. https://www.health.harvard.edu/heart-health/cycling-a-low-impact-exercise-that-helps-the-heart

- Afonso, J., Ramirez-Campillo, R., Moscão, J., Rocha, T., Zacca, R., Martins, A., Milheiro, A. A., Ferreira, J., Sarmento, H., & Clemente, F. M. (2021). Strength Training versus Stretching for Improving Range of Motion: A Systematic Review and Meta-Analysis. Healthcare, 9(4), 427. https://doi.org/10.3390/healthcare9040427

- Johns Hopkins Medicine. (2024). *Osteoarthritis*. Www.hopkinsmedicine.org. https://www.hopkinsmedicine.org/health/conditions-and-diseases/arthritis/osteoarthritis

- Mayo Clinic. (2019). Knee pain - Symptoms and causes. Mayo Clinic. https://www.mayoclinic.org/diseases-conditions/knee-pain/symptoms-causes/syc-20350849

- National Institute on Aging. (2022, November 15). *Osteoporosis*. National Institute on Aging. https://www.nia.nih.gov/health/osteoporosis/osteoporosis

- National Institute on Aging. (2021, January 29). *Four types of exercise can improve your health and physical ability*. National Institute on Aging. https://www.nia.nih.gov/health/exercise-and-physical-activity/four-types-exercise-can-improve-your-health-and-physical

- Johns Hopkins Medicine. (2024). *Osteoarthritis*. Www.hopkinsmedicine.org. https://www.hopkinsmedicine.org/health/conditions-and-diseases/arthritis/osteoarthritis

- United Nations. (2023, January). *World Social Report 2023: Leaving No One Behind In An Ageing World*. UN DESA Publications. https://desapublications.un.org/publications/world-social-report-2023-leaving-no-one-behind-ageing-world

Other Books from Ottie Oz

Visit the Author Page for Ottie Oz for more information and to explore other great books.

amazon.ottieoz.com

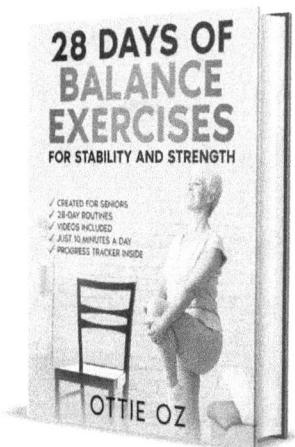

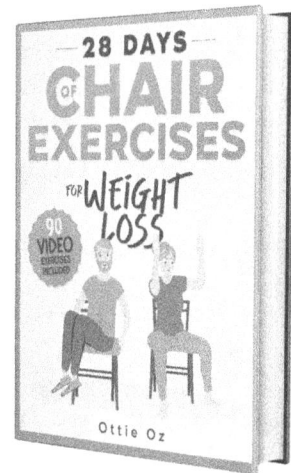

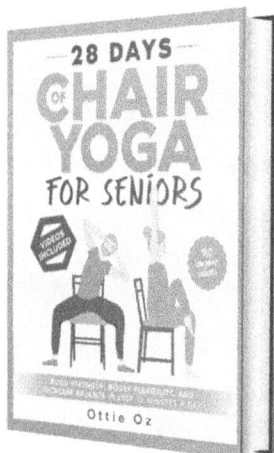

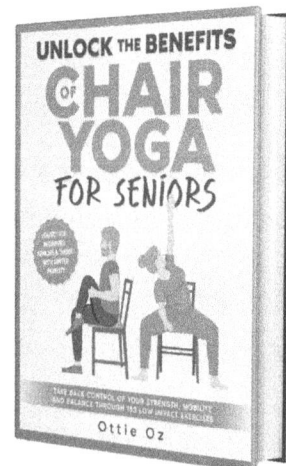